Miguel Attizzani

Cephalometric assessment of individuals with a balanced facial profile

Miguel Attizzani

Cephalometric assessment of individuals with a balanced facial profile

Study carried out on male subjects

ScienciaScripts

Imprint

Cover image: www.ingimage.com

This book is a translation from the original published under ISBN 978-3-330-77019-5.

Publisher:
Sciencia Scripts
is a trademark of
Dodo Books Indian Ocean Ltd. and OmniScriptum S.R.L publishing group

120 High Road, East Finchley, London, N2 9ED, United Kingdom
Str. Armeneasca 28/1, office 1, Chisinau MD-2012, Republic of Moldova, Europe
Managing Directors: Ieva Konstantinova, Victoria Ursu
info@omniscriptum.com

Printed at: see last page
ISBN: 978-620-8-63054-6

CONTENTS

1 INTRODUCTION

The process of diagnosing and planning the treatment of malocclusions has undergone important changes since the introduction of orthodontics as a dental specialty. For many years, achieving satisfactory dental and skeletal cephalometric goals were considered the main objectives to be achieved. However, over time, it was found that in many treatments where these cephalometric goals had been achieved, there was no facial balance or harmony.

Among cephalometric analyses, many do not evaluate the soft tissues of the face or do not relate these tissues to the underlying structures. In addition, most cephalometric analyses use intracranial references which often show significant inter-individual variations, with lower reproducibility than those obtained using extracranial references, and are less suitable for assessing the integumentary profile. Consequently, research using extracranial references and cephalometric analysis of the soft tissues of the face has become more common (ARNETT et al., 1999; SPRADLEY; JACOBS; CROWE, 1981).

There is a growing interest in facial analysis for orthodontic diagnosis and planning. Knowing the relationship between the integumentary tissue of the face and the dento-skeletal structures is of fundamental importance if orthodontic treatments are to provide the best facial aesthetic result, since the orthodontist acts indirectly on the soft tissues when carrying out dental movements or trying to modify the growth of the facial bones.

Diagnostic methodology has favored the evaluation of the soft tissues of the face, either out of idealism or greater knowledge on the part of orthodontists, or in an attempt to satisfy the desires of patients who seek to improve their dental and facial appearance (KIEKENS et al., 2006), or because of the social importance given to a balanced face.

This study evaluated the cephalometric values obtained from individuals with a soft tissue profile considered to be balanced based on subjective visual analysis, and sought to ascertain whether there was any correlation between the harmonious profile and the underlying dentoskeletal structures.

2 LITERATURE REVIEW

2.1 Cephalometric analysis

Radiographic cephalometry is an essential part of the process of diagnosing, planning and evaluating orthodontic, orthopedic and surgical treatments. Most of the cephalometric analyses used in orthodontics prioritize the final positioning of the lower incisors as a reference for achieving success in orthodontic treatment, or even as a guide for defining what other tooth movements will be necessary. However, some researchers have already shown concern about the evaluation of the facial profile and its relationship with dental and skeletal positioning, proposing some references for its evaluation.

Tweed (1944) established cephalometric targets for the final position of the lower incisors, which should be upright on the basal bone at the end of orthodontic treatment, with the aim of providing facial balance and aesthetics, stability of correction, efficiency of the masticatory apparatus and longevity of the tissues. He also related the inclinations of the lower incisors to the facial type of the individuals, with those with predominantly vertical growth having the lower incisors more vestibularized.

Downs (1949) tried to determine the skeletal and dental pattern in individuals with excellent occlusions. To this end, he evaluated lateral teleradiographs of 20 individuals (10 males and 10 females) aged between 12 and 17 years. He concluded that there is a facial pattern representative of the average individual with excellent occlusion. However, he found that some individuals had cephalometric variable values that were quite far from the average, and that skeletal and dental magnitudes could not be assessed in isolation, but as a whole, correlating them with function and aesthetics.

Riedel (1950) carried out a study on 13 individuals after realizing the importance of considering facial aesthetics in the diagnosis and planning of orthodontic treatments. His work was divided into three parts: 1 - A study to verify the concept of a good or bad facial profile; 2 - An analysis of the skeletal and dental tissues of individuals with good and bad facial profiles; 3 - The application of the results in orthodontic diagnosis. He used facial photographs, lateral cephalometric radiographs and plaster models of two groups of patients: 1 - children and adults with clinically assessed normal occlusion; 2 - cases of orthodontically corrected malocclusion. He concluded that there was a relationship between the positioning of the hard and soft tissues, with the anteroposterior relationship between the maxillary and mandibular bone bases, facial convexity and the relationship of the anterior teeth to the face and their respective bone bases having an important influence on the appearance of the soft tissue. According to the author, the more convex the facial profile, the more upright the incisors should be to produce facial harmony. Conversely, in individuals with a straighter skeletal profile, i.e. a small anteroposterior difference between the maxilla and mandible, the incisors could show greater dental protrusion. In general, individuals with smaller facial convexity angles had better facial aesthetics.

Steiner (1953) proposed a cephalometric analysis method to demonstrate the application of cephalometry in the diagnosis and planning of orthodontic treatment, and to facilitate communication with patients' families by quantifying the problems they present. This analysis assesses patients' skeletal and dental patterns. Using measures proposed by other authors and some of his own, he proposed a table that considered factors such as model discrepancy and mechanical procedures to determine the positioning of the incisors at the end of orthodontic treatment. In addition, he advocated calculating cephalometric discrepancy with a diagram based on the ANB angle and the growth of the mentual symphysis. He determined that the ideal measurements of the inclinations of the incisors should be 220 for the upper ones and 250 for the lower ones, in relation to their bone bases.

Holdaway (1956) analyzed changes in the A and B points during orthodontic treatment by means of cephalometric analyses and clinical evaluations. He reported that the ANB angle was a good reference for evaluating and planning orthodontic cases. Although he found that individuals with facial harmony showed variations in the relationships between the bone bases and compensations in the positions of the incisors, he recommended trying to reduce the ANB angle to values close to 2^0 as the aim of orthodontic treatment. He also reported that there could be facial harmony in prognathic and orthognathic individuals, as long as the bone bases did not exceed the limits of dental compensation.

Ricketts (1957) published a study advocating the use of a line called the aesthetic plane or E line, drawn from the most anterior point of the chin to the most anterior point of the nose. The lips were studied in relation to this line, and in individuals with profiles considered disharmonious, the lips projected anteriorly to the aesthetic plane. In individuals with facial harmony, he studied the positioning of the incisors and found that they were positioned 0 to 1mm in front of the A-Pogonion plane and the angle formed by the intersection of this plane with the long axis of the lower incisors was 22^0 to 23^0. Based on this data, he proposed average tooth positioning measures that would provide facial aesthetics.

Riedel (1957) presented a study to determine the dentofacial relationships of a group of 30 women aged between 17 years and 9 months and 21 years and 5 months, selected by the community on the basis of appearance and balance. Photographs were taken of the face and lateral cephalometric radiographs were obtained. Of the sample group, 21 individuals had Class I malocclusion; four had Class II division 1 malocclusion; two had Class II division 1 malocclusion with subdivision and 3 had Class II division 2 malocclusion. He found average values of 3.40 for the ANB angle, inclinations of the upper incisors in relation to the NA line of 17.68^0, and of the lower incisors in relation to the NB line of $23.25^{(0)}$. Riedel then compared these measurements with those obtained in other studies where the sample group consisted of individuals with normal occlusion. He concluded that there were compensatory differences in the values he found, and that the integumentary tissues were related to the underlying dental and skeletal structures.

Burstone (1958) carried out a study with the aim of measuring the facial profile of young, white-skinned adults with faces considered acceptable, so that he could predict skin changes resulting from orthodontic treatment. Lateral teleradiographs of 40 individuals with acceptable faces, as determined by 3 artists from an art school located in Indianapolis, were used. Front and profile photographs were selected. The author concluded that the variability of the integument covering the dental and skeletal tissues was very great, and that it was inappropriate to try to evaluate the face based on dento-skeletal structures.

Subtelny (1959) studied the relationship between skeletal structures and the facial integument. He concluded that the thickness of the integument showed inter-individual variations and that, therefore, the integumentary profile would not always be established by the underlying dentoskeletal structures.

Merrifield (1966) analyzed 120 teleradiographs. Forty were obtained from a sample with normal occlusion that had not undergone orthodontic treatment. Another 40 were from cases treated by Tweed where, according to the author, normal occlusion had been achieved, and finally, 40 radiographs of individuals treated by Merrifield himself, where the planning of the cases took facial aesthetics into account. He then proposed a profile line passing through the soft pogonion and the most prominent point of the upper lip. This line should cross the Frankfurt horizontal plane and would then form the Z angle. The author established ideal values for the Z angle based on the results of this study, which should be 800 (±5) for adults and 78^0(±5) for individuals between 11 and 15 years old. These average values could be used when the FMA, FMIA, IMPA and ANB values are considered normal. According to the author, in individuals with pleasing facial aesthetics, the profile line should tangle the upper and lower lip, or it could be slightly behind this line.

Cox and Van Der Linden (1971) carried out a study using facial profile silhouettes of male and female adults aged between 18 and 20 with white skin, without assessing the type of occlusion of the sample. The profile was evaluated by 10 orthodontists and 10 laypeople, and there was great agreement between the groups. They also found that the individuals with the best facial aesthetics varied more than those proposed in the literature, and that there were a large number of faces with facial harmony and dental malocclusions. The individuals with profiles classified as poor had more convex faces than the others.

Legan and Burstone (1980) proposed a cephalometric analysis of the integument that could be used in patients undergoing orthodontic-surgical treatment. They used a sample of 40 white-skinned adults (20 men and 20 women) aged between 20 and 30 years. The individuals had not been treated orthodontically, had a Class I occlusion and vertical facial proportions within normal limits. To measure the anteroposterior position of the lips, they used a line passing through the subnasal (Sn) and soft pogonion (Pog') points as a reference, measuring the amount of lip protrusion (lips in front of the line) or lip retrusion (lips behind the line). The upper lip should be 3±1mm and the lower lip 2±1mm in front of the Sn-Pog' line. According to the authors, there could be an interlabial gap, and the distance between the upper and lower lip could vary between 2±2mm. At the end of the study, the authors reported that treatment cannot be carried out based solely on cephalometric data of hard tissues, as variations in the integumentary tissue can produce erroneous conclusions about cases.

McBride and Bell (1980) used a "natural" vertical line as a reference to evaluate the aesthetics of the facial profile. This vertical reference line was constructed passing through the subnasal point, perpendicular to a "natural" horizontal line, and was used to assess the relative prominence of the nose, lips and chin. The authors believe that in adult Caucasian individuals, the chin should tangent to this line, and the lips should be slightly in front of it.

Scheideman et al. (1980) studied 24 female and 32 male adults with normal dentoskeletal and integumentary characteristics. All had a chronological age of at least 20 years, an upper and lower facial height ratio of 1:1, Angle Class I, ANB angle between 0 and 4 degrees and no orthodontic treatment or facial surgery. The lateral teleradiographs were taken with the subjects in PNC (natural head position), with the mandible in centric relation and the lips relaxed. As a reference for cephalometric tracings, they used a plane passing through the subnasal point, parallel to the true vertical. They found similar measurements between the genders for the positioning of the chin (-4.5±4.5mm for females and -4.2±3.9mm for males), and greater protrusion for the upper and lower lips in females (1.4±2.0mm in females, 1.0±2.2mm in males and -0.6±2.8mm in females and - 1.4±3.1mm in males respectively).

Spradley, Jacobs and Crowe (1981) evaluated the anteroposterior position of five points on the facial integument below the nose in 25 males and 25 females considered to be young adults. All had pleasant facial profiles and normal sagittal and vertical skeletal relationships. Cephalograms were then obtained with the subjects in their natural head position and a true vertical line. A true horizontal reference plane was constructed perpendicular to the true vertical. From this plane, another was drawn perpendicularly, passing through the subnasal point (Sn), giving it the name subnasal vertical (SnV). The 5 reference points were measured linearly in relation to this vertical line, and the following measurements were found for the male subjects: -1.72±0.78mm for the upper lip sulcus, 1.60±1.68mm for the upper lip, -0.22±1.92mm for the lower lip, -7.94±2.14 mm for the lower lip sulcus and -3.48±2.80mm for the soft pogonion.

Holdaway (1983) believed that orthodontic treatment planning based solely on hard tissue measurements could produce disappointing results. He reported that the first thing to define was what profile we would like to give patients at the end of treatment. Based on this, what therapy would be indicated to achieve these objectives, and if the individual already had facial harmony, what to do to avoid damaging this harmony. He then developed a cephalometric analysis in which the profile of the soft tissues was assessed using the H angle, formed by a tangent to the soft pogonion and upper lip and the Frankfurt horizontal plane. He reported that the greater the facial convexity, the more vestibularized the incisors should be and the greater the H angle should be.

McNamara Jr (1984) proposed a cephalometric analysis with primary application in the diagnosis and treatment planning of patients with facial skeletal discrepancies. He used three samples. The first consisted of teleradiographs taken of children and young people from the Bolton longitudinal study, aged between 6 and 18 years. The second from a group of children and young people aged 6 to 20 with normal occlusion, obtained longitudinally from the Burlington Orthodontic Research Center. The third from a University of Michigan sample of 111 young adults with Class I molar ratios, facial profiles ranging from good to excellent and facial skeletal balance. To arrive at the reference values, he cross-referenced the data from his 3 samples and used them for 9 years, making the adjustments he deemed necessary. He then proposed measures to assess the anteroposterior position of the maxilla and mandible. The reference would be a line perpendicular to the Frankfurt horizontal plane, starting from the nàsio point (N). In adults, this line should ideally pass 1mm behind point A (+1mm) when the maxilla is well positioned in relation to the midface, and from 2mm in front to 4mm behind point Pog (2mm to +4mm) when the mandible is well connected. They also recommended that the effective maxillary length (Co-A) from the condylar point (Co) to the point (A) should be 99.8±6mm for men, and the effective mandibular length (Co-Gn) from the condylar point (Co) to the gnathic point (Gn) should be 132.3±6mm for men.

Park and Burstone (1986) carried out a study to test the effectiveness of using dento-skeletal cephalometric measurements as a clinical tool for predicting and obtaining aesthetic facial results. They studied cephalometric radiographs of 30 adolescent subjects who, at the end of orthodontic treatment, had their lower incisors positioned approximately 1.5mm in front of the A-pogonion plane. For comparison purposes, they used a normal sample of excellent faces (Indiana Sample) of 32 adolescents with an average age of 14.7 years. They then took measurements of the hard and soft tissues. The most important conclusion they reached was that there was a large variation in facial profiles even in cases considered to have been successfully treated, which had achieved the dento-skeletal cephalometric objectives. According to the authors, the results of their work suggest that any average dentoskeletal reference value has questionable validity in producing both adequate facial aesthetics and reproducibility of facial profiles after orthodontic treatment.

Cerci, Martins and Oliveira (1993) evaluated 30 lateral cephalometric radiographs of Brazilians, 15 male and 15 female, aged between 18 and 31 years. All had normal occlusion and a harmonious facial profile. They used a composite of the Steiner and Dows cephalometric analyses for the evaluation, with two aims: to compare the data obtained from the sample made up of Brazilian individuals with that recommended when studying a North American population, and to determine the average standard values for the Brazilian sample. They found statistically significant differences for the cephalometric quantities 1-NA, 1-NB and 1.NA, indicating a typical morphological aspect of dental protrusion. They concluded that these differences and the great variation observed in the sample studied should be taken into account when formulating orthodontic treatment plans for Brazilians.

Czarnecki, Nanda and Currier (1993) published an article in which they studied the perceptions of a balanced facial profile. The authors developed a series of facial profile silhouettes that were evaluated by 545 professionals. They concluded that in males, a straighter profile was preferred, while in females a slightly more convex profile was preferred. The worst profiles were those with an extremely retruded chin or those with very convex faces. They reported that the objectives of orthodontic treatment should be modified, with priority being given to achieving balanced and harmonious facial features rather than seeking treatment goals based on dental and skeletal parameters.

Ozbek and Koklü (1994) evaluated whether the SNA and ANB angle values reflected the amount of maxillary prognathism and intermaxillary relationship with individuals in the natural head position (NHP). They used cephalograms of 106 adults (57 females and 49 males) aged between 19 and 29 with different dental and skeletal characteristics. The authors concluded that there is great variation in individuals with similar facial features, and that the SNA and ANB angles alone did not always represent the integumentary facial pattern of the individuals evaluated.

Epker (1995), dissatisfied with cephalometric assessment as an aid in planning surgical treatments, reported that the main objective should be to make the facial appearance pleasing, not to pay attention to cephalometric standards. He then proposed the use of measurements from different analyses including integumentary, skeletal and dental evaluation. As a reference, he used a line perpendicular to the Frankfurt horizontal plane passing through the subnasal point (SnPerp). He determined that the upper lip should be from 0 to ±2mm in front of this line, the lower lip from -2 to ±2mm and the chin from -4 to ±2mm in relation to the line so that the individuals had a balanced facial profile.

Mantzikos (1998) reported that the study of the subjective concept of beauty should be carried out on different races, as the aesthetic ideal varies in different populations. In his study, he tried to determine the facial profile preferred by a randomly selected sample of 2651 Japanese adults who had lived in the United States for no more than 5 years. With the help of software, 5 different profiles were developed from a photograph. The profiles had the following characteristics: 1 - bimaxillary dentoalveolar retrusion; 2 - retrognathism; 3 -

prognathism; 4 - bimaxillary dentoalveolar protrusion; 5 - orthognathic profile. The evaluators were asked to give marks, with 1 for the most attractive profile and 5 for the least attractive. The order preferred by the evaluators in descending order was: orthognathic profile, bimaxillary dentoalveolar retrusion, bimaxillary dentoalveolar protrusion, retrognathism and prognathism. The author commented that the preference for the orthognathic profile was probably due to advertising, as this profile would not be common to the Japanese.

Nguyen and Turley (1998) evaluated, usingfashion magazines, the changes in the facial profile of young CaucasianCaucasian adults over time, and the profile currently found in this type of publication. The magazines dated from the 1930s to 1995, and 116 photographs of the facial profile were evaluated. The results showed that the male facial profile has changed significantly over time and that these changes have occurred mainly in the lip region. There was a tendency towards an increase in lip protrusion, lip curvature and exposure of lip redness.

Arnett et al. (1999) took lateral teleradiographs of 46 white-skinned, adult models (20 males and 26 females). Before taking the teleradiograph, metal markers were placed on the faces of these individuals at key points defined by the authors. The teleradiographs were taken in the Natural Head Position (NHP). All the patients had untreated Class I occlusions and balanced faces. They then established a true vertical line (TVL) passing through the subnasal point and from there took measurements of the hard and soft tissues. For men, they found the upper lip on average 3.3±1.7mm in front of the TVL line, the lower lip 1±2.2mm in front of the TVL line, the pogonion -3.5±1.8mm behind the TVL line and the tip of the nose 17.4±1.7mm in front of the TVL line. The authors concluded that dento-skeletal factors have a great influence on the facial profile and that the standard values for cephalometric analysis should be different for males and females as there is a great deal of variation between measurements.

Bergman (1999) advocated a facial analysis based on cephalometry because he observed that correcting malocclusions did not always lead to the correction or maintenance of facial features, and that sometimes the appearance of the face worsened after treatment. According to the author, using only cephalometric analyses of dento-skeletal structures to plan treatments can lead to aesthetic problems, especially when the orthodontist tries to predict the facial appearance at the end of treatment, based only on values considered normal for hard tissues. He also stated that the appearance of soft tissue is only partially dependent on the underlying skeletal structures.

Owens et al. (2002) photographically compared the facial appearance of individuals from six racial groups (African-Americans, Caucasians, Chinese, Hispanics, Japanese and Koreans). They found no significant differences between the male and female genders, however, of the 6 measurements used to assess the facial profile, only one (labial-mentonian angle) showed no significant difference between the racial groups.

Bisson and Grobbelaar (2004) compared the lips of models with those of non-models. They used 28 photographs of magazine models, scanned using a *scanner*. As a control group, 14 non-model subjects were selected, of whom digital photographs were taken, then transferred to a computer and evaluated with the same image analysis program used on the models. It was concluded that the height of the upper and lower lip, the angles of the upper and lower lip and the lip thickness were greater in the models than in the control group.

Lopes (2004) radiographically studied 30 Brazilian females with a balanced facial profile, aged between 19 and 31. He used a line parallel to the true vertical, passing through the subnasal point (Sn), called the subnasal vertical (SnV), as a reference for assessing the facial profile. The results were that the nasal projection was 17.2 mm in front of the SnV line, the upper lip 2.1 mm in front of the SnV line, and the lower lip 0.1 mm behind the same line (-0.1 mm). With regard to the projection of the soft pogonion, he found a value of 5.6mm behind the SnV line (-0.56mm). When assessing the skeletal pattern, he found values of 83.1^0 for the SNA angle, 80^0 for SNB, and 3.1^0 for the ANB angle, given by the difference between the first two. The mean value for FNA measurements was 91.7^0, and for FNP 89.8^0. The distance between point A and the N-perp line was 1.8mm, while the distance from point Pog to the N-perp line was 0.3mm. The mandibular plane angle (MFA) had a mean value of 22.7^0. The effective lengths of the maxilla (Co-A) and mandible (Co-Gn) were 94.7mm and 122.3mm respectively. As for tooth positioning, he found 21.8^0 inclination in the upper incisors and 26.9° in the lower incisors.

Correlations between some variables were also studied and the results showed a statistically significant positive correlation between mandibular length and the projection of the lower lip, the projection of the hard pogonion and the soft pogonion, the maxillomandibular relationship and the relationship between the lips, the projection of the upper lip and the soft pogonion, and the projection of the lower lip and the soft pogonion. A statistically significant negative correlation was found between the inclination of the lower incisors and the projection of the lower lip, and the inclination of the lower incisors and the projection of the soft pogonion. The author believes that there is a high degree of variability in the factors that determine facial aesthetics, such as the integument, skeleton and teeth, and that there is an individual compensatory mechanism.

Tukasan et al. (2005) carried out a study to define the cephalometric values of the Tweed Foundation Craniofacial Analysis for a sample of Brazilians. The sample consisted of 211 cephalometric radiographs of individuals aged between 12 and 15 divided into 2 groups: Class II Group with 168 teleradiographs of white-skinned individuals with Class II division 1 of both genders (82 males and 86 females); and the control group, with 43 teleradiographs of individuals with clinically assessed occlusions that were considered excellent, also made up of males (21) and females (22). In the control group, they found a value of 82.47 ± 1.01^{0} for SNA; 80.30 ± 1.08^{0} for SNB; $2.33\pm0.89^{(0)}$) for ANB and $25.12\pm2.74^{(0)}$) for FMA.

Kiekens et al. (2006) conducted a study with laypeople to examine the contribution of measurements routinely used in orthodontic practice to assess facial aesthetics. They used photographs and cephalometric tracings of 64 individuals with Class I, Class II division 1, Class II division 2 and Angle Class III malocclusions. The authors reported that the use of Angle's classification to assess facial aesthetics leads to conflicting results. Furthermore, the measurement of overjet, the ANB angle and the SN-GoMe angle are not decisive in determining the Angle classification or in determining facial aesthetics.

Matoula and Pancherz (2006) analyzed 30 individuals with attractive faces (25 females and 5 males) and 32 with unattractive faces (11 females and 21 males) to try to answer the following question: Is facial beauty related to facial skeletal morphology? In their methodology, they used frontal facial photographs to evaluate facial aesthetics, and lateral cephalometric radiographs to evaluate skeletal and soft tissue features of the face. As the group made up of males with attractive faces was small, it could not be compared to the other groups. When comparing soft tissue profiles without attractive faces between male and female subjects, the male group was found to have greater facial convexity. The authors suggest that in males, a straighter profile is more attractive than a convex one. They concluded that facial beauty in the frontal view is little related to facial skeletal morphology assessed in the lateral view, and that the perception of facial beauty is also related to non-metric factors such as skin color, hair, facial expression and cultural aspects.

Halazonetis (2007) carried out a morphometric evaluation of the shape of the soft tissue profile of the face in order to assess its variability and the differences between male and female individuals. The sample consisted of cephalometric radiographs of 170 orthodontically treated individuals of Greek ethnicity. The classification of malocclusion was not taken into account. In addition, individuals with congenital malformations or syndromes were excluded, as were those with contraction of the labial musculature verified on radiographs and confirmed on facial photographs. The subjects were between 7 and 17 years old and 88 were female, while 82 were male. For the male subjects, he found SNA values of 80.5±3.54^{0}; SNB values of 76.1±3.16^{0}; ANB values of 4.4±2.53^{0}; 1.NA values of 20.5±7.97^{0}; and 1.NB values of 25.6±6.07^{0}.

Scavone Jr. (2008) carried out a study to analyze the anteroposterior integumentary parameters in a sample of white-skinned Brazilian adults and compare them with the values proposed for a sample of white North American adults. They used profile photographs of 59 Brazilians (30 men and 29 women) with normal occlusion and harmonious faces aged between 18 and 30 years. Of the parameters studied, they found the following values for Brazilian males: 15.3±2.1mm for the nasal projection; 2.3±1.8mm for the upper lip projection; 0.0±2.2mm for the lower lip projection and - 4.5±5.1mm for the soft pogonion projection. The only variable analyzed that showed a statistically significant difference between Brazilians and Americans was nasal projection, which was more pronounced in the Americans, on average 2.1mm.

2.2 Natural Head Position (NHP) and Extra-Cranial References

In order to have a standardized and easily reproducible orientation in lateral teleradiographs, the teleradiographs must be taken with the patients in the natural position of the head. The standardization of this position is important because it is independent of the anatomical structures normally used as a reference for teleradiographs, which minimizes errors related to anatomical variations.

Cephalometric analyses by Steiner (1953), Ricketts et al. (1982), McNamara Jr. (1984) and others use the Sela-Nassio line or the Frankfurt horizontal plane as basic reference lines. The variability of the intracranial structures used as reference for tracing these lines can provide erroneous readings, compromising the diagnosis and the orthodontic treatment plan.

Moorrees and Kean (1958), analyzing craniometric studies that used an orientation based on the natural positioning of the head in living beings, tested the hypothesis that this is constant in human beings. According to the authors, confirmation of this hypothesis would mean the possibility of using an extracranial reference, called the True Vertical (VER), in cephalometric studies. In order to assess the reproducibility of the NHP, cephalometric studies were carried out on female patients aged between 18 and 20, separated into two groups. Group 1, containing 66 students, was radiographed twice, with a one-week interval between the first and second radiographs, and the individuals were instructed to assume the Natural Head Position. Group 2, containing 61 individuals, was also x-rayed twice, with the same time interval, but in this group, the individuals had their head position corrected before the recording. The standard deviation of the head position in the 66 students in the first group was 2.05^0, and in the second 1.540. The smaller variation for the second group was due to the correction of the Natural Head Position. With this, they verified the relative constancy of the Natural Head Position and consequently the possibility of using the True Vertical to determine the reliability of the intracranial reference lines. Based on this, they evaluated the range of variation of some intracranial cephalometric references, including the Saddle-Nassus line and the Frankfurt Horizontal Plane. To do this, they used the radiographs of group 2. The comparison between the references showed a variation of 3.55° to 6.69° in these intracranial references, which was greater than the variation in the recording of the position of the head. They concluded that the method described for obtaining cephalometric radiographs in the Natural Position of the Head and the use of a True Vertical line as a reference is more reliable than the routine use of some lines such as the Frankfurt Horizontal Plane or the Saddle-Nassus line.

Lundstrom and Lundstrom (1995) carried out a study to determine the reliability of the Frankfurt Plane as a reference line using the lateral cephalometric tracings of 79 English children aged 12, whose records were taken in the Natural Head Position. The angles formed by the Frankfurt Horizontal Plane and the Saddle-Nasio line in relation to the True Vertical were analyzed. According to the analysis of the results obtained, no statistically significant variations were found between the Frankfurt Horizontal Plane and the Saddle-Nose line. As a horizontal reference, the use of a line related to the Natural Position of the Head is indicated, which corresponds to the most reliable reference for use in cephalometric analysis.

According to Rino Neto et al. (2002), the intracranial reference lines S-N and the Frankfurt horizontal plane show greater variability than the extracranial lines. The authors also report that the NCP record shows statistically significant reproducibility, corroborating its use in obtaining lateral cephalometric radiographs.

Rino Neto, Freire Maia and Paiva (2003) recommended a method for obtaining the natural position of the head oriented to the lateral cephalometric radiographs used in the Post-Graduate Orthodontics course at the University of São Paulo School of Dentistry. Individuals should stand with their feet 10 cm apart and tilt their heads up and down, decreasing the amplitude of the movement with each series, until they feel that the natural balance of the head has been achieved. The patient is then instructed to look at the image of their own eyes reflected in an oval mirror positioned in front of them. The olives are inserted into the cartilaginous *tragus* to prevent the head from rotating. The non-tissue positioner is then adapted to the non-tissue point region to stabilize the head in a vertical direction. The final position is checked by an experienced professional, and if they notice any kind of deviation, this should be corrected. The true vertical line is represented by a metal chain with a weight at its lower end. It is positioned close to the anterior edge of the film holder frame, so that its image appears in front of the contour of the soft tissue profile. Finally, the

X-ray beam is fired and the radiograph is taken.

Madsen, Sampson and Townsend (2008) compared the reproducibility obtained using the true horizontal line (HOR) with that obtained using some intracranial reference planes that are less commonly used than the Frankfurt planes and the Sela-Nassio line and which, according to the authors, had not yet been studied, such as the Krogman-Walker (KW) line, the neutral horizontal axis, the foramen magnum line and the posterior maxillary plane. They used a sample made up of 38 female and 19 male subjects, of whom facial photographs and lateral teleradiographs were taken with the subjects in the natural position of the head. The results showed that the intracranial planes with the best reproducibility were twice as good as the reproducibility obtained using the true horizontal line (HOR).

3 JUSTIFICATION

The use of intracranial references and analyses based mainly on hard tissue can lead to planning errors and situations where skeletal and dental cephalometric values do not match what is observed in the integumentary profile. Given the great importance of facial aesthetics today, comparing soft tissue cephalometric values with hard tissue cephalometric values using an extracranial reference may highlight the need to use dento-skeletal information with caution, bearing in mind that the aesthetic objective cannot be neglected in favor of correcting malocclusion.

4 OBJECTIVES

To evaluate the following characteristics using lateral cephalograms of male subjects with a balanced facial profile:

- The nasal projection, labia and soft pogonion in relation to the vertical subnasal line.
- The skeletal position of the maxilla and mandible in relation to the skull base.
- The inclination of the upper and lower incisors in relation to their respective bone bases.
- The correlations between integumentary, dental and skeletal structures.

5 MATERIAL AND METHODS

5.1 Material

Lateral cephalometric radiographs were taken of 25 young Brazilian males, white skinned, aged between 18 and 33 years, with an average age of 22.3 years, living in the state of São Paulo (Appendix A), from a pre-selection of 467 individuals.

5.2 Methods

Students from undergraduate and postgraduate courses at the University of São Paulo were invited to take part in the study. The research subjects were recruited via an e-mail sent to all the students at the University of São Paulo, by posters put up at all the bus stops in the Armando Salles de Oliveira University City, by a radio program on Radio USP, and by small lectures in the teaching units, explaining the importance of the work and urging the students to take part. From a group of 467 volunteers, digital photographs were taken of the faces of 120 people. The photographs were taken from the frontal and right profile views using a digital camera (Nikon Coolpix 990) (Figure 5.1 and 5.2). The subjects were photographed standing, in the natural position of the head oriented in relation to the horizon line, with teeth occluded and lips relaxed. Names and contact telephone numbers were then recorded.

The photographs were transferred to a computer (Toshiba Satellite A65-S126) and evaluated by four experienced orthodontists who voted "yes" to accept and "no" to discard each photograph according to the following criteria:

- Balance of the lower third of the face - the upper lip was in front of the lower lip, which in turn was in front of the chin;
- Lip sealing;
- White skin;
- Brazilians.

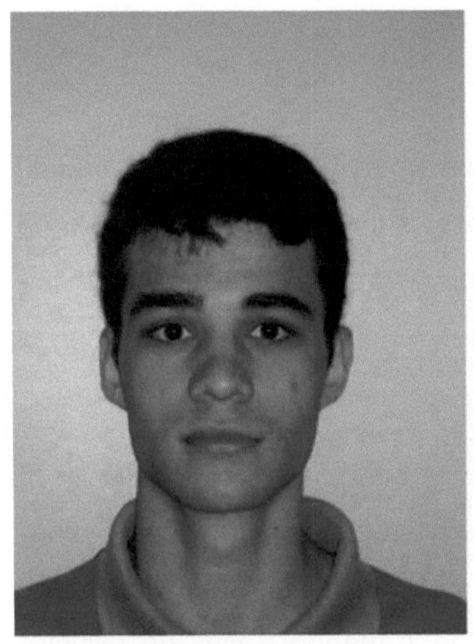

Figure 5.1 - Front photograph

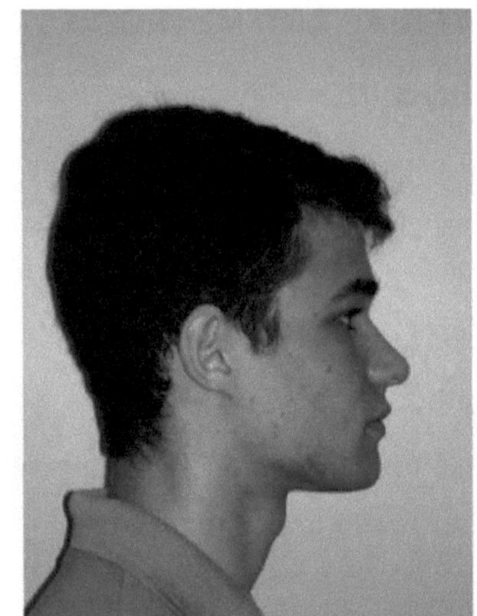

Figure 5.2 - Profile shot

The photograph was selected when there was unanimity among the evaluators in relation to the above-mentioned items.

After selection, the individuals were contacted by telephone and called to FOUSP's Department of Orthodontics and Pediatric Dentistry to sign an informed consent form, have their occlusions assessed (Appendix B) and undergo the photography and teleradiography procedures.

5.2.1 Photographic method

Frontal and right profile photographs were taken with the subjects standing in a natural head position oriented in relation to the horizon line, with their teeth occluded and lips relaxed. When the subjects' heads were not in the correct position, they were instructed by the operator to assume a natural oriented position. An oval mirror was positioned in front of the subjects so that they could look into their own eyes, serving as an orientation of the horizon line. A metal wire with a ruler at the end was positioned in front of the subjects to act as a reference for the true vertical (Figure 5.4). The camera used was a Canon Rebel Assault 2000, set to the M function with a speed of 60 and an aperture of 22. The film used was Kodak with the Asa 100 specification.

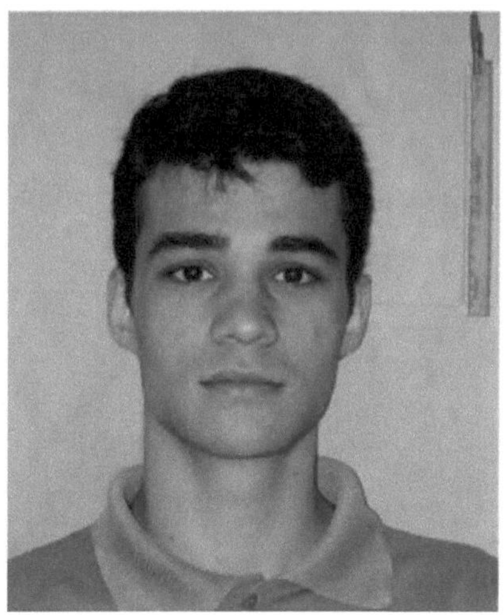

Figure 5.3 - Front photograph

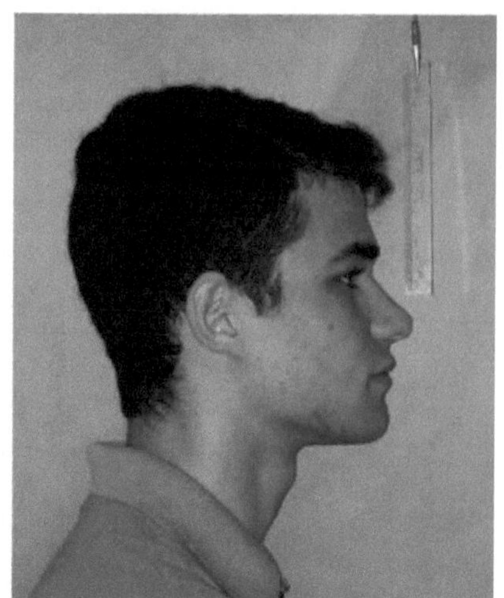

Figure 5.4 - Profile shot

5.2.2 Method for obtaining lateral cephalometric radiographs

The X-ray machine used was the Panoura 10 - CSU, PA 810 model from Yoshida Dental, MFG Co Ltda, Tokyo-Japan, with a working regime of 85 kVp and 10 mA with an exposure time of 1.2 seconds. The subjects were given radioprotection material and instructed to keep their lips at rest and their teeth in maximum habitual intercuspation, according to the natural head position technique. They were instructed to stand in an upright, relaxed position, looking at their own eyes in the mirror. In this position, the pupils are centered in the middle of the eyes, defining the line of sight or true horizontal. When it became clear that the posture of the subjects' heads was unnatural, they were instructed to assume the natural "oriented" position. A plumb bob was attached to the X-ray machine representing the true vertical according to the criteria described by Lundstrom and Lundstrom (1992, 1995), Lundstrom et al. (1995) and Rino Neto, Freire-Maia and Paiva (2003) (Figure 5.5). At a distance of 1.52m from the X-ray source to the object, an aluminum filter was used to highlight the integumentary profile of the face. Kodak X-ray films were used,

18 x 25 cm in size and mounted in a chassis (Figure 5.6). The lateral cephalometric radiograph was then taken (Figure 5.7). All the teleradiographies were taken by the same operator.

Development was carried out mechanically using an *Air Techniques* model A/T 2000 automatic processor (Figure 5.8), with development criteria based on the manufacturer's internal parameters.

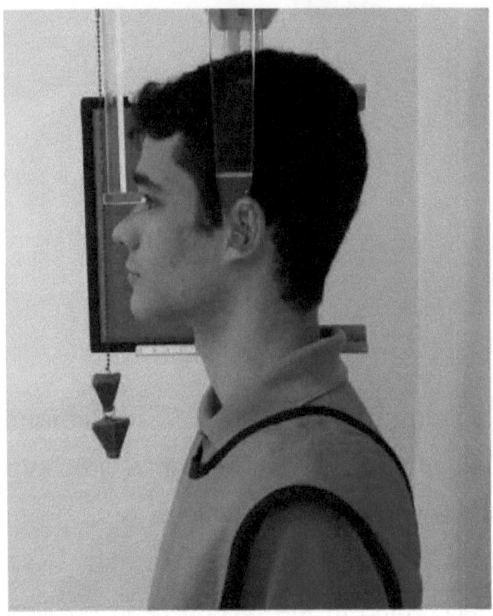

Figure 5.5 - Individual positioned in the oriented PNC

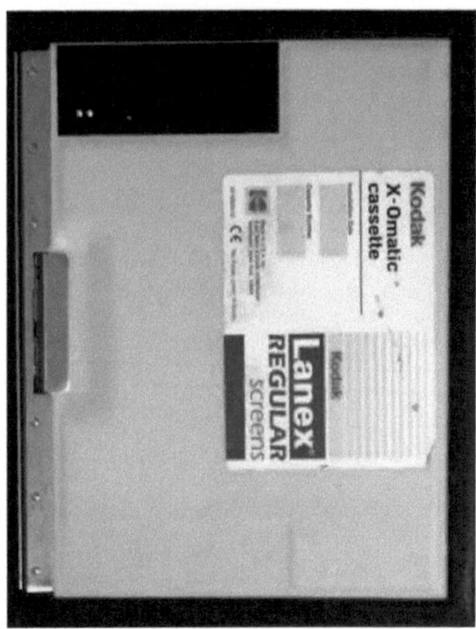

Figure 5.6 - Radiographic chassis

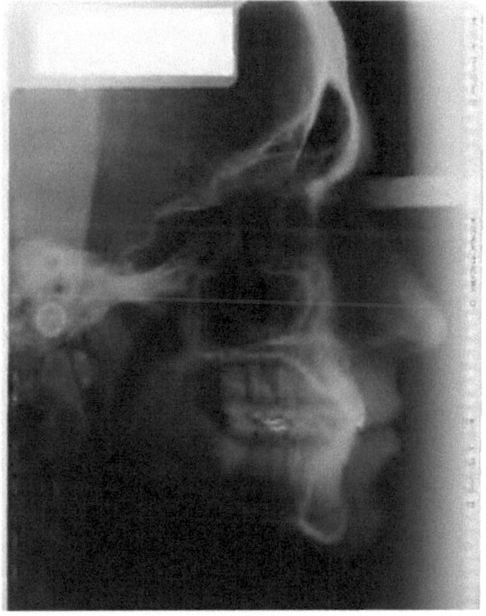

Figure 5.7 - Lateral X-ray

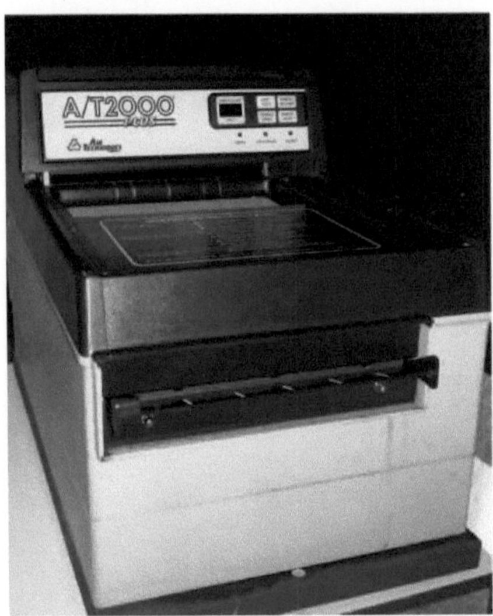

Figure 5.8 - Automatic processor

5.2.3 Method for obtaining cephalometric tracings

The teleradiographs were digitized using a scanner (HP Scanjet 6100c) and transferred to the Radiocef Studio 2 *software.* A program tool was used to calibrate the size of the scanned images. In order to increase the accuracy of marking the cephalometric points, tools were used in the Radiocef program® which allowed the use of geometric magnification resources and changes in the contrast of the radiographic images, which helped in marking the points. A cephalometric analysis specific to the research was developed, using the resource called MIXCEF.

The cephalometric points were then marked on each of the radiographs, and the program automatically measured the desired linear and angular distances.

5.2.3.1 Cephalometric points used (Figure 5.9)

- Point N (nâsio): Most anterior point of the frontonasal suture;
- Orbital point: Lowest point on the contour of the orbits;
- Point S (saddle): Point located in the center of the image of the Turkish saddle;

- Ponto Po (pório): Uppermost point in the image of the external auditory canal;
- Co point (condyle): Most superior and posterior point of the mandibular head contour;
- Go point: The most inferior and posterior point of the mandibular angle. It is determined by the bisector of the angle formed by the tangents to the lower edge of the mandibular body and the posterior edge of the ramus;
- Me (mentonian) point: Lowest point on the contour of the mentual symphysis;
- Point Gn (gnàtio): The most anterior and inferior point of the mental symphysis, demarcated by the projection of the bisector of the angle formed between the facial plane (NP) and the mandibular plane (Go-Me);
- Pog point: the most anterior point of the mandibular symphysis;
- Point A (subspinal): deepest point of the anterior concavity of the maxilla, between the anterior nasal spine and the prosthium;
- Point B (supramentonian): deepest point of the anterior contour of the mentual symphysis, between the infradental and pogonionic points;
- Point Ais (apex of the upper incisor): midpoint of the root apex of the upper incisors;
- Point Iis (incisal of the upper incisor): midpoint of the incisal edge of the upper incisors;
- Point Aii (lower incisor apex): midpoint of the root apex of the lower incisors;
- Point Iii (incisal of the lower incisor): midpoint of the incisal edge of the lower incisors;
- Pog' point (pogonion-line): the most anterior point of the integumentary mentual region;
- Ls point (upper lip): the most anterior point of the upper lip contour;

- Li point (lower lip): the most anterior point of the lower lip contour;
- Point Sn (subnasal): point where the upper lip and the base of the nose intersect;
- Pn (pronasal) point: most prominent point of the nose on the integument;
- Point V1 (vertical 1): point on the true vertical line;
- Point V2 (vertical 2): randomly located at a point below point V1 on the true vertical line.

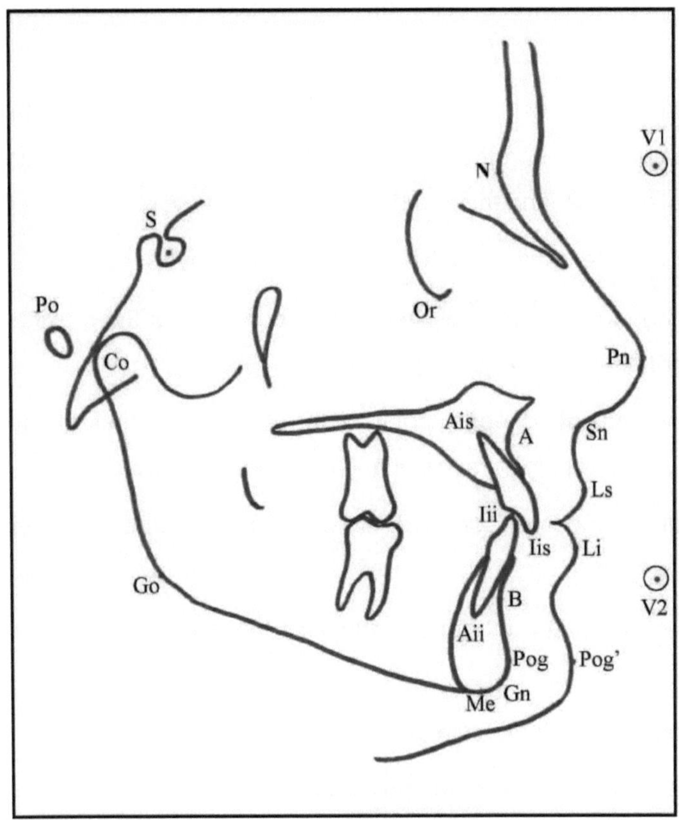

Figure 5.9 - Anatomical drawing and points used to obtain the cephalometric tracing

5.2.3.2 Lines and planes used (Figures 5.10, 5.11, 5.12, 5.13 and 5.14)

- Line S-N: determined by joining points S and N;

- Frankfurt Horizontal Plane: determined by joining the points Po and Or;
- Mandibular plane: determined by the junction of the Go and Me points;
- N-A line: determined by joining points N and A;
- N-B line: determined by joining points N and B;
- N-Pog line: determined by joining points N and Pog;
- Co-A line: determined by joining points Co and A;
- Co-Gn line: determined by joining the Co and Gn points;
- True Horizontal Line: line perpendicular to the true vertical that passes through point S.
- True Vertical Line: line passing through points V1 and V2;
- SnV line: line perpendicular to the true horizontal passing through point Sn;
- Long axis of the maxillary central incisor: line passing through points Iis and Ais;
- Long axis of the lower central incisor: line passing through points Iii and Aii;
- N-Perp line: line perpendicular to the Frankfurt horizontal plane passing through point N.

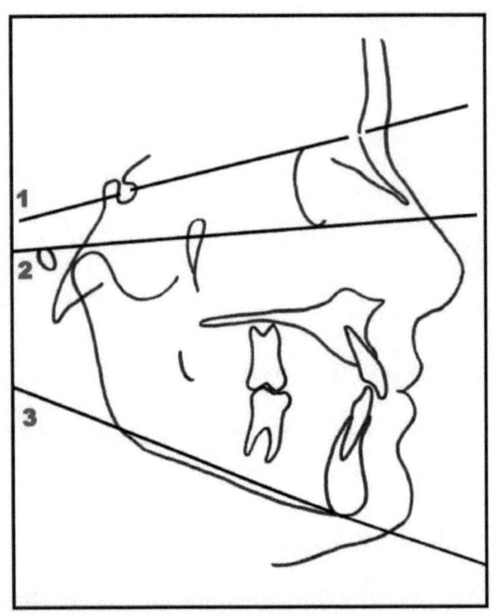

Figure 5.10 - S-N line (1), Frankfurt horizontal plane (2) and mandibular plane (3)

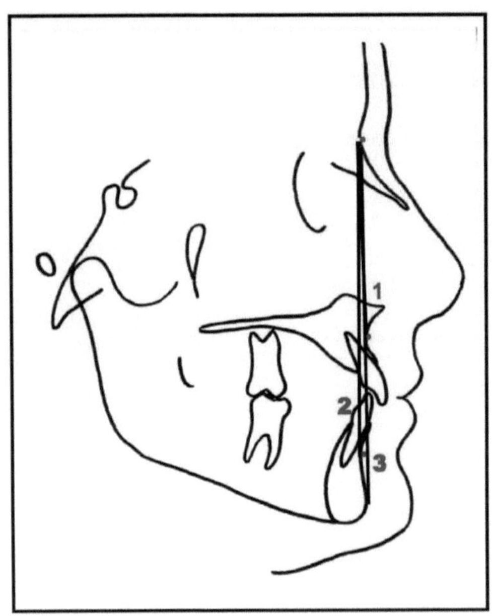

Figure 5.11 - NA Line (1), NB Line (2) and Npog Line

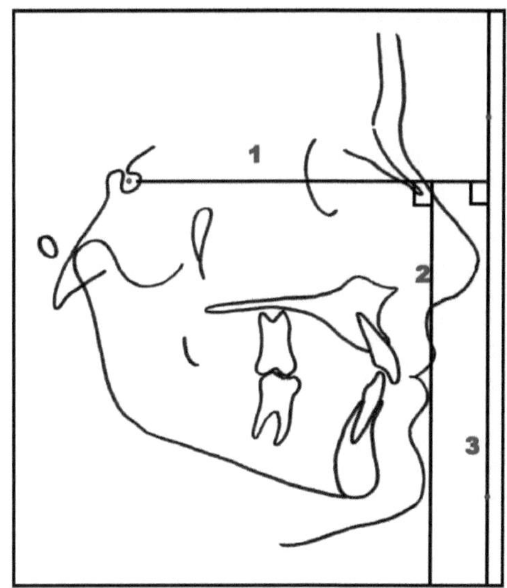

Figure 5.12 - True Horizontal Line (1), SnV Line (2) and True Vertical Line (3)

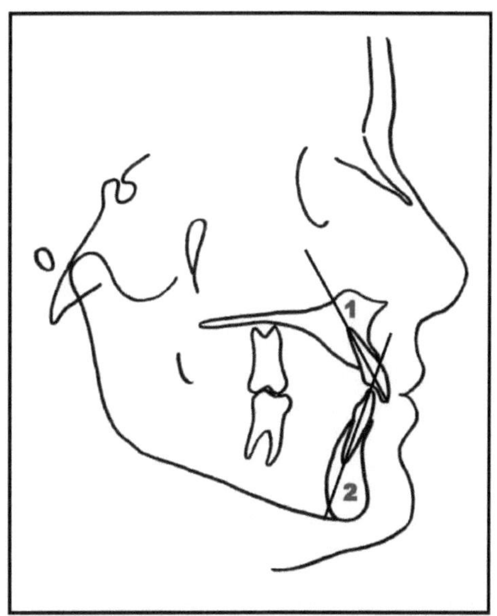

Figure 5.13 - Long axis of upper (1) and lower (2) incisors

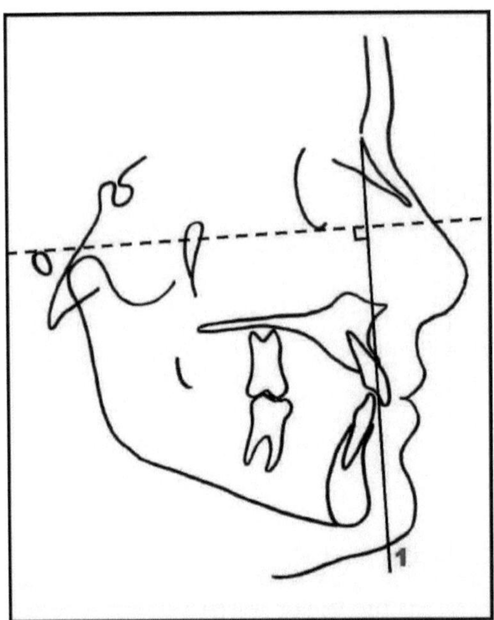

Figure 5.14 - N-perp line (1)

5.2.3.3 Cephalometric skin measurements (Figures 5.15 and 5.16)

- SnV-Pn: distance between line SnV and point Pn;
- SnV-Ls: distance between the SnV line and the Ls point;
- SnV-Li: distance between the SnV line and the Li point;
- SnV-Pog': distance between the SnV line and the Pog' point;
- LsLi-HV: distance from point Ls to point Li projected on the true horizontal line.

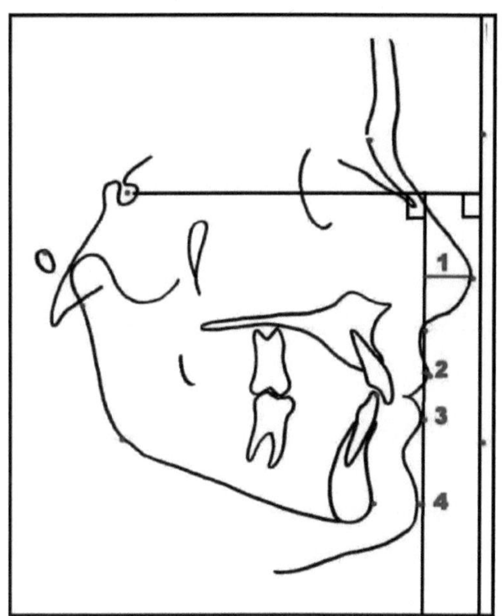

Figure 5.15 - SnV-Pn distance (1), SnV-Ls distance (2), SnV-Li distance (3) and SnV- distance (4).

Pog' (4)

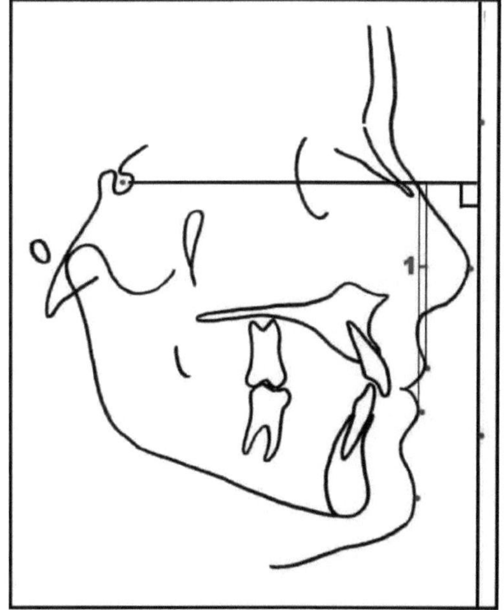

Figure 5.16- LsLi-HV distance (1)

5.2.3.4 Cephalometric skeletal measurements (Figures 5.17, 5.18, 5.19, 5.20 e 5.21)

- SNA: angle formed by the S-N and N-A lines;
- SNB: angle formed by lines SN and NB;
- ANB: angle formed by lines NA and NB;
- FNA: angle formed by the horizontal plane ofFrankfurt e a line NA;
- FNP: angle formed by the horizontal plane ofFrankfurt e a line NPog;
- FMA: angle formed by the horizontal plane ofFrankfurt e a line Go-Me line;
- Co-A: distance from point Co to point A;
- Co-Gn: distance from point Co to point Gn;
- A-Nperp: distance from point A to the N-perp line;
- Pog-Nperp: distance from the Pog point to the N-Perp line.

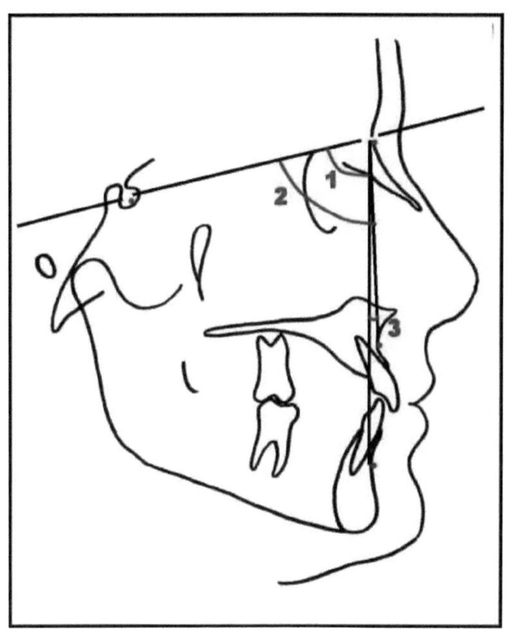

Figure 5.17 - Angles SNA (1), SNB (2) and ANB (3)

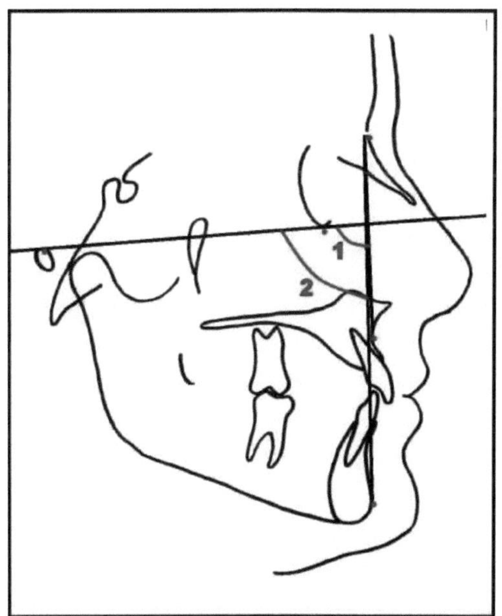

Figure 5.18 - FNA (1) and FNP (2) angles

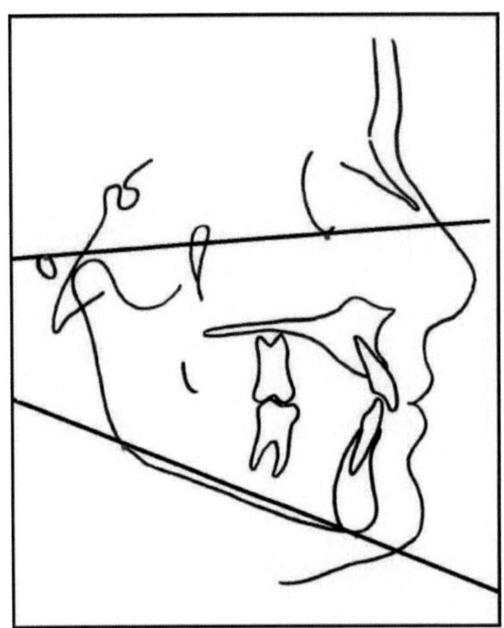

Figure 5.19 - FMA angle

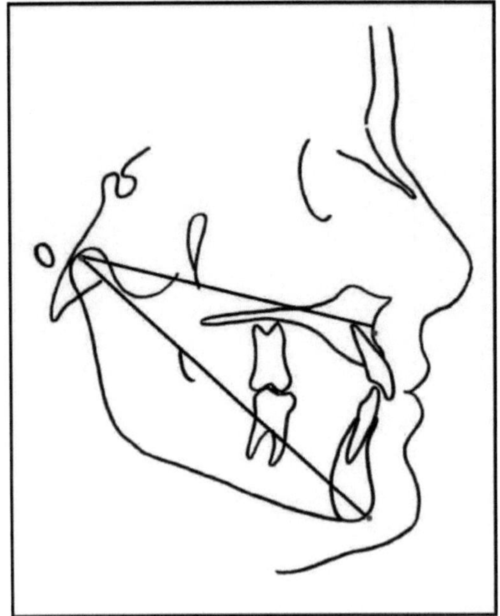

Figure 5.20 - Co-A and Co-Gn distance

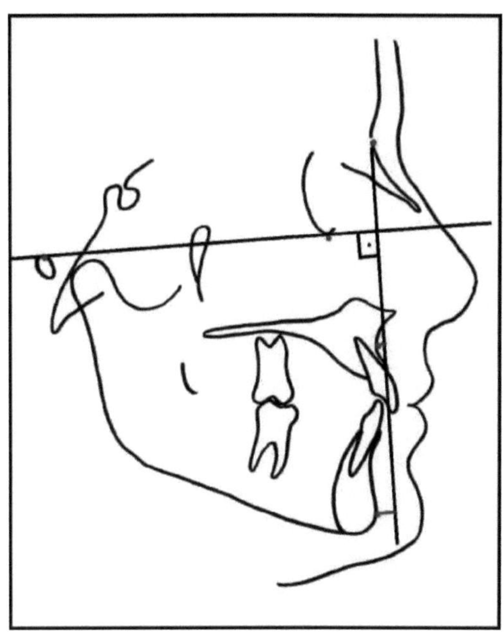

Figure 5.21 - A-Nperp and P-Nperp distances

5.2.3.5 Dental cephalometric measurements (Figure 5.22 and 5.23)

- 1.NA: angle formed by the intersection the long axis of the incisors

with the NA line;

- 1.NB: angle formed by the intersection the long axis of the incisors

with the NB line.

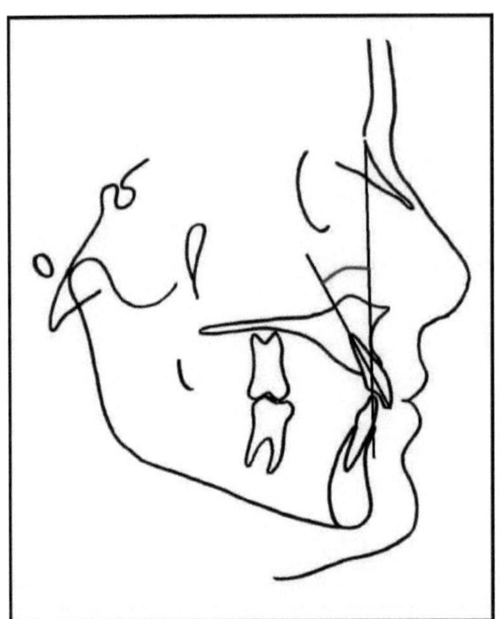

Figure 5.22 - Angle 1.NA

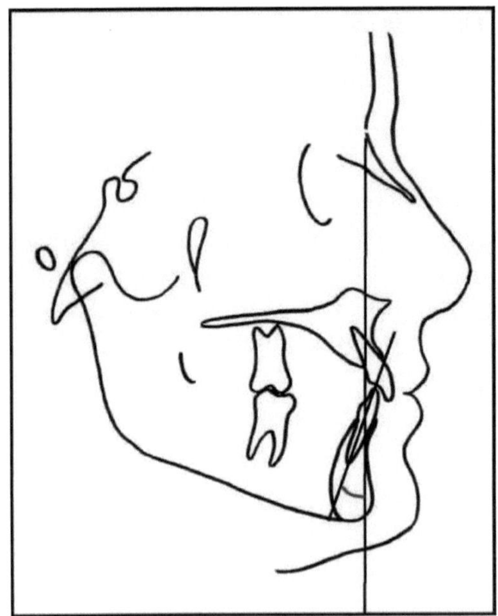

Figure 5.23 - Angle 1.NB

1.1.1.6 Cephalogram used (Figure 5.24)

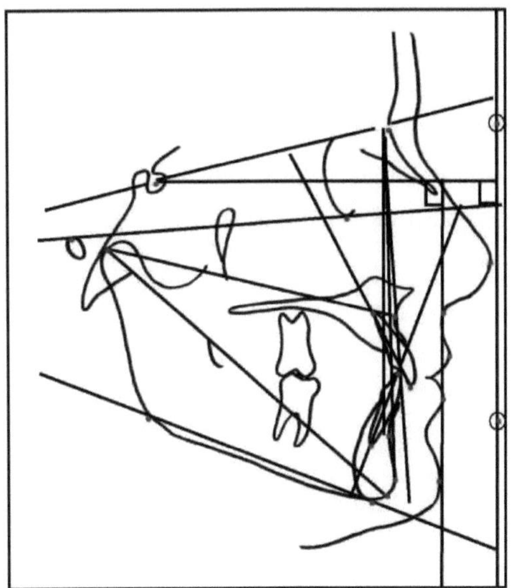

Figure 5.24 - Cephalogram used with orientation lines and pianos, cephalometric measurements tegumentary, skeletal and dental measurements

5.2.4 Statistical methods

To answer the objective of the study, the normal distribution of the observed variables was first tested using the Kolmogorov-Smirnov and Shapiro-Wilk tests (CONOVER, 1980). The mean, standard deviation, median, minimum, maximum and normality interval (BUSSAB; MORETTIN, 1987) were calculated for each variable. Pearson's correlation matrix was calculated between all the variables (BUSSAB; MORETTIN, 1987). The tests were carried out at a 5% significance level.

5.2.5 Method error

To assess the error of the cephalometric measurement method, 10 lateral cephalometric radiographs were taken after 60 days, and all the cephalometric points used were marked by the same operator. The error of the method was checked using intraclass correlation (FLEISS, 1986) and Dalhberg's formula

(DALHBERG, 1940), as follows:

$$\sqrt{\frac{\sum d^2}{2n}}$$

where d is the difference between the two measurements and n is the number of individuals studied.

6 RESULTS

The distribution of the variables was considered normal (p>0.05), according to the Kolmogorov-Smirnov and Shapiro-Wilk tests (Table 6.1).

Table 6.1 Kolmogorov-Smirnov and Shapiro-Wilk tests

	Kolmogorov-Smirnov			**Shapiro-Wilk**		
Variables	statistics	gl	p	statistics	gl	p
FNA	0,73	25	0,656	0,96	25	0,461
SNA	0,42	25	0,994	0,98	25	0,941
SNB	0,72	25	0,681	0,96	25	0,492
ANB	0,64	25	0,814	0,96	25	0,445
1.NA	0,79	25	0,563	0,94	25	0,152
1.NB	0,48	25	0,974	0,97	25	0,564
FMA	0,54	25	0,932	0,96	25	0,412
FNP	0,60	25	0,863	0,98	25	0,838
Co-Gn	0,62	25	0,843	0,98	25	0,812
Co-A	0,56	25	0,909	0,97	25	0,695
SnV-Ls	0,51	25	0,958	0,96	25	0,482
SnV-Li	0,51	25	0,957	0,97	25	0,752
LsLi-HV	0,44	25	0,990	0,96	25	0,493
SnV-Pog'	0,53	25	0,942	0,99	25	0,984
SnV-Pn	0,63	25	0,825	0,97	25	0,692
A-Nper	0,70	25	0,710	0,97	25	0,636
Pog-Nperp	0,56	25	0,914	0,98	25	0,910

Table 6.2 shows that the observed measurements have very close to 100% agreement for all measurements (intraclass correlation > 0.9) with the exception of the FMA measurement (intraclass correlation = 0.49). Dalhberg's formula showed that, for none of the variables, the calculated errors exceeded 1mm or 1 degree, with the exception of measurements 1.NA and 1.NB.

Table 6.2 - Method error

Variable	Intraclass correlation	Dalhberg's formula
FNA	0,98	0,57
SNA	0,97	0,76
SNB	0,98	0,64
ANB	0,81	0,96
1.NA	0,97	1,03
1.NB	0,95	1,15
FMA	0,49	0,86
FNP	0,97	0,44
Co-Gn	0,99	0,64
Co-A	0,98	0,91
SnV-Ls	0,93	0,40
SnV-Li	0,93	0,47
LsLi-HV	0,88	0,41
SnV-Pog'	0,97	0,39
SnV-Pn	0,92	0,63
A-Nperp	0,97	0,64
Pog-Nperp	0,97	0,96

$p<0,05$

Table 6.3 shows the mean, standard deviation, median, minimum and maximum values for the skin measurements studied. The upper lip was on average positioned in front of the SnV line, while the lower lip and chin were positioned behind the SnV line, with the chin positioned behind the lower lip. The nasal projection was 17.94±2.07mm in front of the SnV line. The average horizontal distance between the upper and lower lips was 2.24±1.05mm.

Table 6.3 - Mean, standard deviation, median, minimum and maximum for skin measurements

Variable	Average	DP	Median	Minimum	Maximum	N
SnV-Ls	2,20	1,29	2,32	0,13	4,52	25
SnV-Li	-0,24	1,61	-0,41	-3,24	3,49	25
SnV-Pog'	-5,95	2,59	-6,36	-11,55	-0,04	25
SnV-Pn	17,94	2,07	17,83	14,35	22,44	25
LsLi-HV	2,44	1,05	2,38	0,09	4	25

SD - standard deviation; N - sample number

Table 6.4 shows the mean, standard deviation, median, minimum and maximum values for the skeletal measurements studied.

Table 6.4 - Mean, standard deviation, median, minimum and maximum for skeletal measurements

Variable	Average	DP	Median	Minimum	Maximum	N
FNA	89,94	4,04	90,61	81,64	96,94	25
SNA	84,80	5,12	84,95	74,62	94,6	25
SNB	82,82	4,11	83,39	75,24	91,77	25
ANB	1,81	2,51	1,76	-2,77	6,38	25
FMA	22,91	3,18	22,92	17,02	31,74	25
FNP	90,58	2,65	90,97	84,62	95,89	25
Co-Gn	137,70	7,56	136,79	122,63	152,91	25
Co-A	103,33	6,43	104,4	91,55	115,98	25
A-Nper	0,00	4,36	-0,66	-7,49	9,5	25
Pog-Nperp	-1,31	5,73	-2,03	-13,07	11,03	25

SD - standard deviation; N - sample number

Table 6.5 shows the mean, standard deviation, median, minimum and maximum values found for the dental measurements.

Table 6.5 - Mean, standard deviation, median, minimum and maximum for dental measurements

Variable	Average	DP	Median	Minimum	Maximum	N
1.NA	25,87	6,76	26,24	13,71	38,22	25
1.NB	27,22	4,26	27,42	16,86	34,29	25

SD - standard deviation; N - sample number

Table 6.6 shows the correlations found between the variables, where one of them was necessarily an integumentary variable. No statistically significant correlations were found between dental and skin variables.

Table 6.6 - Main correlations between the measurements studied.

Variables	r	p
AMF and LsLi-HV	0,400	0,048*
SnV-Ls and SnV-Li	0,764	<0,001***
SnV-Li and SnV-Pog'	0,700	<0,001***
LsLi-HV and SnV-Pog'	-0,632	0,001**
FNA and SnV-Pog'	-0,406	0,044*
SnV-Li and LsLi-HV	-0,598	0,002**
SnV-Pog' and Pog-Nperp	0,543	0,005**

*p<0.05; **p<0.01; ***p<0.001

7 DISCUSSION

The mass media, the cult of beauty and its association with success are factors that influence the search for a pleasing appearance, and dentistry plays an important role in pursuing this goal.

Orthodontic, orthopedic and orthodontic-surgical treatments can correct dental malpositions, modify growth, alter the positioning of bone bases and the contour of the soft tissues that make up the face. Given that there is conflicting information between skeletal and dental cephalometric values and integumentary appearance, it is not prudent for orthodontic treatments, which should provide facial balance and adequate occlusion, to be planned based simply on skeletal and dental measurements. We believe that a diagnosis and treatment plan based on an analysis "from the outside in", correlating the integumentary structure with intracranial characteristics, allows professionals to establish objective treatment criteria. Teleradiographs taken in lateral view with the subjects in the natural position of the oriented head (LUNDSTROM; LUNDSTROM, 1992; 1995; LUNDSTROM et al, 1995; RINO NETO; FREIRE-MAIA; PAIVA, 2003) using extracranial references for clinical and radiographic assessment (ARNETT et al., 1999; SPRADLEY; JACOBS; CROWE, 1981; SCHEIDEMAN et al., 1980; MADSEN; SAMPSON; TOWNSEND, 2008) are fundamental to the use of this protocol. However, there may be differences in preference for certain facial features, due to ethnic differences and cultural backgrounds (MANTZIKOS, 1998; MATOULA; PANCHERZ, 2006), changes in facial preference that occur over time (NGUYEN; TURLEY, 1998), as well as differences between the male and female genders (BERGMAN, 1999). The search for a better understanding of the interrelationship between extracranial and intracranial structures in Brazilian individuals motivated this research.

For better understanding, the discussion has been divided into five topics: integumentary pattern, skeletal pattern, dental pattern, correlations and final considerations.

7.1 Skin pattern

7.1.1 Upper lip

In this study, the average value found for the positioning of the upper lip in relation to the SnV line was 2.20±1.29mm. Scheideman et al. (1980) found 1±2.2mm in their sample of male subjects. However, these authors did not choose a sample with ideal facial features, which could partly explain this difference. Spradley et al. (1981), also studying 25 males, found 1.60±1.68mm for the projection of the upper lip in relation to the SnV line, a mean value also lower than that found in the present study. In this study's sample, the minimum value found for the upper lip projection was 0.13mm. This value is close to the mean value minus standard deviation (-0.08mm) found by Spradley et al. (1981), while the maximum upper lip projection value in the present study was 4.52mm, further away from the mean value plus standard deviation (3.28mm) found by Spradley et al. (1981). In this study, one of the inclusion criteria was that the upper lip was positioned in front of the lower lip. In Spradley et al. (1981), the authors only mention that individuals with a good facial profile were selected for the study. It is likely that the accuracy of the inclusion criteria and the ancestry of the sample may have influenced the cephalometric values found. Arnett et al. (1999) found upper lip projection values of 3.3±1.7mm when studying a sample of American individuals. These values are higher than those found in this study. This can also be explained by the fact that they used a sample made up of photographic models, whose lips are thicker than the "normal population" (BISSON; GROBBELAAR, 2004). Scavone Jr. et al. (2008), studying profiles based on photographic images obtained from a sample made up of individuals of Brazilian nationality, found 2.3±1.8mm for the upper lip projection, a value very close to that of the present study.

7.1.2 Lower lip

For the projection of the lower lip, a value of -0.24±1.61mm was found. This value is higher than that found by Scheidman et al. (1980) (1.4±3.1mm) and lower than those of Spradley et al. (1981) (-0.22±1.92mm), Arnett et al. (1999) (1±2.2mm) and Scavone Jr. et al. (2008) (0±2.2mm). In all the studies, the standard deviation values are higher than the average values found, which means that there is a high degree of variability in the positioning of the lower lip. It is also notable that in individuals with "ideally" balanced profiles, the lower lip was always positioned behind the upper lip. In view of this finding, and in the absence of values for the distance between the upper and lower lip in the sagittal plane in males, we investigated the distance projected on a true horizontal line (LsLi-HV). The mean value found was 2.44±1.05mm. Lopes (2004) studied this variable for a female sample and found a value of 2.3±1mm, very close to that of this male sample.

As in his work, this variable was the one with the lowest standard deviation, corroborating the assertion that in balanced faces, the upper lip is always positioned in front of the lower lip, and that they are closely related to each other.

7.1.3 Soft pogonium

As for the projection of the soft pogonion in relation to the SnV line, the average values found in this study were -5.95±2.59mm. McBride and Bell (1980) recommended 0mm as the ideal value for positioning the soft pogonion in relation to the SnV line, i.e. the pogonion should be tangential to the SnV line. Scheideman et al. (1981) found values of -4.5±4.5mm to be ideal. Commenting on the work by McBride and Bell (1980), Scheideman et al. (1980) stated that the discrepancy in values in their studies was related to the individual preference of each maxillofacial surgeon. Spradley et al. (1981) found values of -3.48±2.80mm for the soft pogonion in relation to the SnV line in male subjects. Later, Arnett et al. (1999) studied 20 male models and found values of -3.5±1.8mm. Lopes (2004) using a sample made up of females, found -5.6±3.3mm and Scavone Jr. et al. (2008), 4.5±5.1mm for males. The samples selected by Americans seem to tend towards a straighter soft tissue profile, with a greater projection of the chin, which may denote a type of preference dictated by ethnic difference and/or the evaluators' own perception. In research carried out on Brazilian population groups, there seemed to be greater acceptance of a slightly more convex profile.

7.1.4 Nasal projection

Nasal projection also seems to be subject to variation in harmonic male faces. While Scheidman et al. (1980) found an average value of 21.5±1.8mm, the value found in this study was 17.94±2.07mm. This value is close to the 17.4±1.7mm recommended by Arnett et al. (1999). Scavone Jr. et al. (2008) studied a group of Brazilian males and found a nasal projection value of 15.3±2.1mm. Nasal projection was not used as one of the criteria for selecting this sample. However, it is clear that the shape of the nose, its projection and the privileged position it occupies on the face play an important role in facial balance. Orthodontists don't treat nasal disharmonies, but they must be aware of the interrelationship between the nose, upper lip, lower lip and chin. This knowledge is a prerequisite for understanding the normal range of the facial profile.

7.2 Skeletal pattern

7.2.1 Maxilla

To evaluate the maxilla, we used the SNA, FNA, Co-A and A-Nperp measurements.

The SNA defines the anteroposterior positioning of the maxilla in relation to the skull base. In the present study, a value of 84.80 ± 5.12^0 was found for this measurement. The average reference value proposed by Riedel (1950) was 82^0. Scheideman et al. (1980) found values of 82.4 ± 3.9^0, close to those found by Cerci, Martins and Oliveira (1993) in a sample of Brazilians with normal occlusion and a harmonious facial profile of 82.23 ± 2.82^0.

Tukasan et al. (2005) found values of 82.38^0 for a group of male patients with excellent occlusion, and 83.67^0 for a group of individuals with Class II. In this study, the type of malocclusion according to Angle's classification (1907) was not taken into account. From the values found for SNA (84.80±5.12^0), applying the standard deviation, it could be said that some individuals in the sample had maxillary protrusion or retrusion in relation to the skull base, if the values recommended by Riedel (1950) of SNA=82±2^0 were taken into account. However, this statement is not significant for diagnosis and planning, since all the individuals had a balanced soft tissue profile. This is a warning not to focus on cephalometric measurements in isolation, given the known variability of the intracranial structures used to obtain cephalometric measurements.

The average value found for the FNA measurement was 89.94±4.04^0, i.e. within the average recommended in the literature (90±3^0) (RICKETTS et al.,1982).

The A-Nperp and Co-A measurements were evaluated together. In this study, since the value found for A-Nperp was 0mm, it could be said, taking into account the value recommended by McNamara Jr. (1984) of 1mm, that the maxilla was slightly retruded in relation to the skull base. When the mean value for the effective length of the maxilla was evaluated (103.33±6.43mm), it was found to be within the normal range. In relation to the effective length of the maxilla (Co-A), it should also be evaluated in relation to the effective length of the mandible (Co-Gn), and according to McNamara Jr. (1984), a difference between 30 and 33 mm is considered normal. The data found in this sample (Co-A=103.33±6.43mm and Co-Gn=137.70±7.56mm) showed that the difference between the values for the effective lengths of the maxilla and mandible were within normal limits.

7.2.2 . Mandible

The SNB, FNP, Co- Gn and Pog-Nperp measurements were used to assess the mandible.

The SNB measurement assesses the anteroposterior positioning of the mandible in relation to the skull base. The value found was 82.82 ± 4.11^{0}, slightly higher than the average value (80^{0}) recommended by Riedel (1950), Scheideman (1980) of $80.9^{(0)}$), Cerci, Martins and Oliveira (1993) of $80.73\pm2.80^{(0)}$) Tukasan (2005) of $80.29^{(0)}$) and Halazonetis (2007) of 76.1 ± 3.16^{0}. The value of the ANB angle, which reflects the maxillo-mandibular relationship, showed a mean value of 1.810. This value is close to that found by Scheideman (1980) of 1.6^{0} and Cerci, Martins and Oliveira (1993) of $1.50^{(0)}$) and slightly lower than that recommended by Riedel (1950) with 2^{0} and that found by Tukasan (2005) with 2.240. It is considerably lower than that found by Halazonetis (2007) 4.4 ± 2.53^{0}, who, however, did not select the individuals in his study based on facial balance, but rather on the diversity of profiles, which may partly explain this difference.

The value found for the FNP measure (90.58 ± 2.58^{0}) was within the average values recommended by Downs (1949). This value was also close to that found by Lopes (2004) in a sample made up of females (89.86±2.050).

The anteroposterior positioning of the mandible in relation to the skull base, expressed by the cephalometric quantity Pog-Nperp, showed a value of -1.31±5.73mm. McNamara Jr. (1984) proposed values of between -2 and 2mm for this magnitude. It should be noted that, based on the minimum and maximum values found for all the variables relating to the positioning of the maxilla and mandible, it can be said that they showed a high degree of variation. Because of this high variability, it can be said that more important than being close to the pre-established targets for skeletal values is harmony between the craniofacial and integumentary components for each individual.

Evaluation of the FMA angle revealed a mean value of 22.91 ± 3.18^{0}. The range of values indicating a normal facial growth pattern for this angle proposed by Tweed (1954) is 210 to 290. Of the 25 individuals studied, only 3 had values lower than 20^{0}, and only 1 had more than 29^{0} (APPENDIX G).

7.3 Dental pattern

The inclination values of the upper incisors in relation to the NA line and the lower incisors in relation to the NB line were analyzed.

7.3.1 Upper incisors

The average value found for the inclination of the upper incisors was 25.87 ± 6.76^{0}. Cerci, Martins and Oliveira (1993) analyzed a sample of Brazilian males with harmonious facial profiles and found mean values of 24.27 ± 4.71^{0}, very close to those in this study. These values are higher than those recommended by Steiner (1953), with 22^{0} and by Scheideman et al. (1980) who found a value of 21 ± 6^{0} for male individuals. Riedel (1957) found a value of 17.60 for the inclination of the upper incisors, and Lopes (2004) 21.8 ± 5.6^{0}. However, although they studied samples of individuals with balanced faces, only females were assessed. Furthermore, as in this study, the authors did not take into account the type of malocclusion, which may also explain the fact that in this study we found a minimum value of 13.710 and a maximum value of 38.220 (APPENDIX G) for the inclination of the upper incisors.

7.3.2 Lower incisors

For the inclination of the lower incisors in relation to their bone base, the mean value found was 27.22 ± 4.26^{0}, slightly higher than the $25^{(0)}$) recommended by Steiner (1953), 23.2(0) by Riedel (1957), 22.3±4.8(0) by Scheideman et al. (1980) and $23.77\pm3.80(^{0})$ by Cerci, Martins and Oliveira (1993). Although the sample used in this study was made up of males, the average values found were close to those found in the sample made up of females studied by Lopes (2004) with an average value of 26.9 ± 4.1^{0}. It is also important to note that we found very discrepant values for the inclination of the lower incisors in relation to their bone bases, even in individuals with balanced faces. The minimum inclination value was 16.860 and the maximum was 34.29^{0}, which may be partly associated with the variability of anterior facial height, which was not the subject of this study. However, it was found that in the sample there were 3 individuals with FMA values lower than 200, and 1 with a value higher than 29^0. Given the high variability of the inclination of the lower incisors at their respective bone bases, using them as a reference in the search for facial balance may not be the most appropriate method.

7.4 Correlations

No statistically significant correlations were found between skeletal and dental magnitudes (APPENDIX F). Although significant correlations were found between skeletal magnitudes (APPENDIX F), between integumentary magnitudes (APPENDIX F), between skeletal and dental magnitudes (APPENDIX F), and between skeletal and integumentary magnitudes (APPENDIX F), the discussion was limited to correlations in which integumentary magnitudes were involved.

The main positive correlations found were:

- When FMA increased in value, there was an increase in the distance between the upper and lower lips (LsLi-HV) ($p=0.048$).

With an increase in the value of the mandibular plane angle (FMA), we can expect clockwise rotation of the mandible and a more posterior positioning. With the mandible slightly more retruded, the horizontal distance between the upper and lower lips tends to increase.

- Anteriorization of the upper lip (SnV-Ls) was directly related to anteriorization of the lower lip (SnV-Li) ($p<0.001$).

This result is related to one of the criteria for selecting the sample, which was that the upper lip should be discreetly in front of the lower lip in order to achieve harmony in the facial profile.

- The positioning of the lower lip and soft pogonion in relation to the SnV line also showed a directly proportional correlation ($p<0.001$).

The more anteriorized the lower lip was, the more anteriorized the soft pogonion was.

- The projection of the pogonium in relation to the perpendicular Nàsio line (Pog- Nperp) and of the pogonium in relation to the SnV line (SnV-Pog') showed a positive correlation ($p<0.001$).

The soft pogonion followed the projection of the skeletal structure, becoming more anteriorized.

The main negative correlations found were:

- Between the FNA value and SnV-Pog' ($p=0.044$).

This can be explained by the fact that the anteriorization of the maxilla may have led to anterior projection of the Sn point, and consequently the distance between the soft chin (Pog') and the SnV line would also have increased.

- When there was an increase in the value of the cephalometric quantity SnV-Li, there was a decrease in the distance between the upper and lower lips (LsLi-HV) ($p=0.002$). This was expected, since if the lower lip is more anteriorized, the distance between it and the upper lip will be smaller.

- Between the distance between the upper and lower lips (Ls-Li-HV) and the projection of the soft pogonion (SnV-Pog') ($p=0.001$).

This correlation showed that the greater the distance between the upper and lower lips, the more retruded the soft pogonion was in relation to the SnV line.

7.5 Final considerations

The acceptance of a facial profile as balanced does not seem to be related to an exact average cephalometric value, but to a composition of factors between the tissues that make up the face. In this study, it became clear that the use of pre-established averages should only serve as a reference, since cephalometric assessments do not always correspond to what is visualized on people's faces. The numerical value of skeletal and dental cephalometric measurements should be considered, especially if they are representative of the individual's face. Among the objectives of orthodontic treatment, there is always the concern of achieving facial balance. Therefore, orthodontic diagnosis and the treatment plan must be carried out taking into account individual characteristics, cultural aspects, facial analysis, study models, the patient's complaint and the possibilities and limitations of the therapies used.

8 CONCLUSIONS

It can be concluded that in the sample studied:

- The average nasal projection was 17.94mm, the upper lip 2.20mm, the lower lip -0.24mm and the soft pogonion -5.95mm in relation to the vertical subnasal line.
- The mean values for the positioning of the maxilla and mandible in relation to the skull base were 84.80^0 and 82.82^0 respectively.
- The average inclinations of the upper and lower incisors in relation to their bone bases were 25.87^0 and 27.22^0 respectively.

The most statistically significant positive correlations were:

- Mandibular plane angle (FMA) and the distance between the upper and lower lips (LsLi-HV) ($p=0.048$);
- The projection of the upper lip (SnV-Ls) and lower lip (SnV-Li) ($p<0.001$);
- A projection of the lower lip (SnV-Li) and the soft pogonion (SnV-Pog') ($p<0.001$);
- A pogonium projection (Pog-Nperp) and soft pogonium (SnV-Pog') ($p=0.005$).

The most statistically significant negative correlations were:

- The projection of the maxilla and the projection of the soft pogonion ($p=0.044$);
- The projection of the lower lip and the distance between the upper and lower lips ($p=0.002$),
- The distance between the upper and lower lips and the projection of the soft pogonion ($p=0.001$).

REFERENCES*

Angle EH. Malloclusion of the teeth. 7th ed. Philadelphia: S. S. White Manufacturing; 1907.

Arnett GA, Jelic JS, Kim J, Cummings DR, Beress A, Worley CM, et al. Soft tissue cephalometric analysis: Diagnosis and treatment planning of dentofacial deformity. Am J Orthod Dentofacial Orthop 1999;116(3):239-53.

Bergman RT. Cephalometric soft tissue facial analysis. Am J Orthod Dentofacial Orthop 1999;116(4):373-89.

Bisson M, Grobbelaar A. The esthetic properties of lips: A comparison of models and nonmodels. Angle Orthod 2004;74(2):162-6.

Burstone CJ. The Integumental Profile. Am J Orthod 1958;44(1):1-25.

Bussab WO, Morettin PA. Basic Statistics. 4a ed. Sao Paulo: Atual; 1987.

Cerci V, Martins JES, Oliveira MA. Cephalometric standards for White Brazilians. Int J Adult Orthod Orthognath Surg 1993;8(4):287-92.

Conover, WJ. Practical nonparametric statistics. 2nded. New York: Wiley; 1980.

Cox NJ, Van Der Linden FPGM. Facial harmony. Am J Orthod 1971;60:175-84.

Czarnecki ST, Nanda RS, Currier GF. Perceptions of a balanced facial profile. Am J Orthod Dentofacial Orthop 1993;104(2):180-7.

Dahlberg G. Statistical methods for medical and biological students. New York, Interscience; 1940.

Downs WB. Variation in facial relationship: their significance in treatment and prognosis. Am J Orthod 1949;19(3):145-55.

Epker BN. Dentofacial deformities: integrated orthodontic and surgical correction. 2nd ed. St. Louis: Mosby; 1995.

Fleiss JL. The design and analysis of clinical experiments. New York: Wiley; 1986.

Halazonetis DJ. Morphometric evaluation of soft-tissue profile shape. Am J Orthod Dentofacial Orthop 2007;131(4):481-9.

Holdaway RA. Changes in relationship of points A and B during orthodontic treatment. Am J Orthod 1956;42:176-93.

* According to Vancouver Style. Journal abbreviations according to MEDLINE database.

Holdaway RA. A soft-tissue cephalometric analysis and its use in orthodontic treatment planning. Part I. Am J Orthod 1983;84(1):1-28.

Kiekens RMA, Maltha JC, van't Hof MA, Kuijpers-Jagtman AM. Objective Measures as Indicators for Facial Esthetics in White Adolescents. Angle Orthod 2006;76(4):551-6.

Legan HI, Burstone CJ. Soft tissue cephalometric analysis for orthognathic surgery. J Oral Surg 1980;38(10):744-51.

Lopes KB. Tegumentary, skeletal and dental evaluations of the facial profile [Master's dissertation]. Sao Paulo: USP School of Dentistry; 2004.

Lundstrom A, Lundstrom F. Natural head position as a basis for cephalometric analysis. Am J Orthod Dentofacial Orthop 1992;101(3):244-7.

Lundstrom A, Lundstrom F. The Frankfort horizontal as a basis for cephalometric analysis. Am J Orthod 1995;107(5):537-40.

Lundstrom A, Lundstrom F, Lebret LML, Moorrees CFA. Natural head position and natural head orientation: basic considerations in cephalometric analysis and research. Eur J Orthod 1995;17(2):111-20.

Madsen DP, Sampson WJ, Townsend GC. Craniofacial reference plane variation and natural head position. Eur J Orthod 2008;30(5):532-40.

Mantzikos T. Esthetic soft tissue profile preferences among the Japanese population. Am J Orthod Dentofacial Orthop. 1998;114(1):1-7.

Matoula S, Pancherz H. Skeletofacial Morphology of Attractive and Nonattractive Faces. Angle Orthod 2006;76(2):204-10.

McBride KL, Bell WN. Chin surgery. In: Bell WH, Proffit WR, White RP. Surgical correction of dentofacial deformities. Philadelphia: WB Saunders Company; 1980. chap 14. p. 121179.

McNamara Jr. JA A method of cephalometric evaluation. Am J Orthod 1984;86(6):449-69.

Merrifield LL. The profile line as an aid in critically evaluating facial esthetics. Am J Orthod 1966;52(11):804-22.

Moorrees CF, Kean MR. Natural head position: a basic consideration in the interpretation of cephalometric radiographs. Am J Phys Anthropol 1958;16(2):213-34.

Nguyen DD, Turley PK. Changes in the Caucasian male facial profile as depicted in fashion magazines during the twentieth century. Am J Orthod Dentofacial Orthop 1998;114(2):208-17.

Ozbek MM, Koklü AY. Extracranial versus intracranial references in individual cephalometric analysis. Br J Orthod 1994;21(3):259-63.

Owens EG, Goodacre CJ, Loh PL, Hanke G, Okamura M, Jo K, et al. A Multicenter Interracial Study of Facial Appearance. Part 1: A Comparison of Extraoral Parameters. Int J Prosthod 2002;15(3):273-82.

Park YC, Burstone CJ. Soft-tissue profile-Fallacies of hard-tissue standards in treatment planning. Am J Orthod 1986;90(1):52-62.

Ricketts RM. Planning treatment on the basis of the facial pattern and an estimate of its growth. Angle Orthod 1957;27(1):14-37.

Ricketts RM, Roth RJ, Chaconas SJ, Schulhof R J, Engel GA. Orthodontic diagnosis and planning: their roles in preventive and rehabilitative dentistry. Denver: Rocky Mountain Company; 1982. v.1. p. 133.

Riedel RA. Esthetics and its relation to orthodontic therapy. Angle Orthod 1950;20:168-78.

Riedel RA. An analysis of dentofacial relationships. Am J Orthod 1957;43(2):103-19.

Rino Neto J, Paiva JB, Freire-Maia BA, Miasiro Junior H, Attizzani MF, Crivello Junior O. Evaluation of the Reproducibility of the Natural Head Position: Radiographic Study. Ortodontia 2002;35(4):55-68.

Rino Neto J, Freire-Maia BA, Paiva JB. Method of recording the natural position of the head for obtaining lateral cephalometric radiographs - Considerations and importance of the method in orthodontic-surgical diagnosis. Rev Dental Press 2003;8(3):61-71.

Scavone Jr H, Zahn-Silva W, Valle-Corotti KM, Nahàs ACR. Soft Tissue Profile in White Brazilian Adults with Normal Occlusions and Well-Balanced Faces. Angle Orthod 2008;78(1):58-63.

Scheideman GB, Bell WB, Finn RA, Reisch JS. Cephalometric analysis of dentofacial normals. Am J Orthod Dentofacial Orthop 1980;78(4):404-20.

Spradley FL, Jacobs JD, Crowe DP. Assesment of the anteroposterior soft-tissue contour of the lower facial third in the ideal young adult. Am J Orthod 1981;9(3):316-25.

Steiner CC. Cephalometrics for you and me. Am J Orthod 1953;39(10):729-55.

Subtelny JD. A longitudinal study of soft tissue facial structures and their profile characteristics defined in relation to underlying skeletal structures. Am J Orthod 1959;45:481-507.

Tukasan PC, Magnani MBBA, Nouer DF, Nouer PRA, Neto JSP, Garbui IU. Craniofacial analysis of the Tweed Foundation in Angle Class II, division 1 malocclusion. Braz Oral Res 2005;19(1):69-75.

Tweed CH. Indications for the extraction of teeth in orthodontic procedure. Am J Orthod 1944;30:405-28.

Tweed CH. The Frankfort-mandibular incisor angle (FMIA) in orthodontic diagnosis, treatment planning and prognosis. Angle Orthod 1954;24(3):121-69.

APPENDIX

APPENDIX A - Age of research subjects

Research subject	Age
RLBA	23 years old
MPS	24 years old
GRD	21 years old
KBL	33 years old
FFS	22 years old
RAB	23 years old
FS	23 years old
RAR	22 years old
PPF	19 years old
PSJ	22 years old
CNG	20 years
RR	19 years old
RFS	24 years old
PZ	22 years old
CCC	22 years old
AFPS	22 years old
CPT	21 years old
BS	28 years old
CSO	20 years
LSL	23 years old
RBC	22 years old
FCO	20 years
EDL	18 years old
JCM	22 years old
DBS	24 years old

APPENDIX B - Classification of malocclusions, assessment of previous orthodontic treatment and approximate time taken to complete orthodontic treatment for the group studied

Individual	Malocclusion	Treatment Orthodontic	Completion of treatment
RLBA	Cl I	Yes	10 years
MPS	Cl I	Yes	3 years
GRD	Cl I	Yes	1 month
KBL	Cl II	Yes	8 years
FFS	Cl I	Yes	2 years
RAB	Cl III	Yes	9 years
FS	Cl I	Yes	2 years
RAR	Cl I	Yes	5 years
PPF	Cl	Yes	3 years
PSJ	Cl I	Yes	7 years
CNG	Cl I	No	
RR	Cl I	Yes	4 years
RFS	Cl I	No	
PZ	Cl I	No	
CCC	Cl I	Yes	6 years
AFPS	Cl I	No	
CPT	Cl I	Yes	8 years
BS	Cl I	No	
CSO	Cl I	Yes	7 years
LSL	Cl I	No	
RBC	Cl I	No	
FCO	Cl I	No	
EDL	Cl I	No	
JCM	Cl I	No	
DBS	Cl I	Yes	8 years

APPENDIX C - Correlations between variables

Variables	r	p
FNA and SNA	-0,731	<0,001***
FNA and SNB	-0,486	0,014*
FNA and ANB	-0,707	<0,001***
FNA and 1.NA	0,631	0,001*
FNA and 1.NB	-0,152	0,469
FNA and FMA	0,187	0,370
FNA and FNP	0,761	<0,001***
FNA and Co-Gn	0,030	0,887
FNA and Co-A	-0,213	0,306
FNA and SnV-Ls	-0,277	0,180
FNA and SnV-Li	-0,202	0,333
FNA and SnV-Pog'	-0,406	0,044*
FNA and LsLi-HV	-0,034	0,873
FNA and SnV-Pn	0,229	0,272
FNA and A-Nper	-0,997	<0,001***
FNA and Pog-Nperp	-0,761	<0,001***
SNA and SNB	0,891	<0,001***
SNA and ANB	0,685	<0,001***
SNA and 1.NA	-0,394	-0,051
SNA and 1.NB	0,310	0,131
SNA and FMA	-0,135	0,519
SNA and FNP	-0,504	0,010*
SNA and Co-Gn	0,032	0,878
SNA and Co-A	0,173	0,408
SNA and SnV-Ls	0,300	0,145
SNA and SnV-Li	0,293	0,156
SNA and LsLi-HV	-0,075	0,721
SNA and SnV-Pog'	0,330	0,107
SNA and SnV-Pn	-0,337	0,100
SNA and A-Nperp	0,732	<0,001***
SNA and Pog-Nperp	0,499	0,011*
SNB and ANB	0,309	0,132
SNB and 1.NA	-0,059	0,780
SNB and 1.NB	0,088	0,676

SNB and FMA	-0,055	0,796
SNB and FNP	-0,543	0,005**
SNB and Co-Gn	0,019	0,929
SNB and Co-A	-0,085	0,686
SNB and SnV-Ls	0,210	0,314
SNB and SnV-Li	0,304	0,139
SNB and LsLi-HV	-0,201	0,336
SNB and SnV-Pog'	0,380	0,061
SNB and SnV-Pn	-0,317	0,122
SNB and A-Nperp	0,480	0,015*
SNB and Pog-Nperp	0,538	0,006*
ANB and 1.NA	-0,734	<0,001***
ANB and 1.NB	0,499	0,011*
ANB and FMA	-0,156	0,456
ANB and FNP	-0,156	0,457
ANB and Co-Gn	0,093	0,658
ANB and Co-A	0,493	0,012*
ANB and SnV-Ls	0,344	0,092
ANB and SnV-Li	0,126	0,548
ANB and LsLi-HV	0,228	0,272
ANB and SnV-Pog'	0,082	0,696
ANB and SnV-Pn	-0,173	0,408
ANB and A-Nperp	0,718	<0,001***
ANB and Pog-Nperp	0,155	0,460
1.NA and 1.NB	-0,222	0,286
1.NA and FMA	0,224	0,282
1.NA and FNP	0,237	0,253
1.NA and Co-Gn	-0,319	0,120
1.NA and Co-A	-0,614	0,001*
1.NA and SnV-Ls	-0,157	0,453
1.NA and SnV-Li	0,039	0,854
1.NA and LsLi-HV	-0,253	0,222
1.NA and SnV-Pog'	-0,112	0,592
1.NA and SnV-Pn	-0,141	0,502
1.NA and A-Nperp	-0,647	<0,001***
1.NA and Pog-Nperp	-0,238	0,252

1.NB and FMA	0,099	0,637
1.NB and FNP	0,320	0,119
1.NB and Co-Gn	-0,138	0,512
1.NB and Co-A	0,268	0,195
1.NB and SnV-Ls	0,307	0,135
1.NB and SnV-Li	0,122	0,560
1.NB and LsLi-HV	0,191	0,360
1.NB and SnV-Pog'	-0,182	0,384
1.NB and SnV-Pn	-0,083	0,694
1.NB and A-Nperp	0,159	0,448
1.NB and Pog-Nperp	-0,327	0,111
FMA and FNP	0,139	0,507
AMF and Co-Gn	0,104	0,621
AMF and Co-A	-0,203	0,330
FMA and SnV-Ls	0,361	0,077
FMA and SnV-Li	0,020	0,926
AMF and LsLi-HV	0,400	0,048*
FMA and SnV-Pog'	-0,114	0,588
FMA and SnV-Pn	-0,120	0,567
AMF and A-Nperp	-0,199	0,340
AMF and Pog-Nperp	-0,141	0,502
FNP and Co-Gn	0,023	0,914
FNP and Co-A	0,146	0,486
FNP and SnV-Ls	-0,146	0,485
FNP and SnV-Li	-0,196	0,349
FNP and LsLi-HV	0,112	0,593
FNP and SnV-Pog'	-0,577	0,004**
FNP and SnV-Pn	0,171	0,415
FNP and A-Nperp	-0,747	<0,001***
FNP and Pog-Nperp	-0,999	<0,001***
Co-Gn and Co-A	0,757	<0,001***
Co-Gn and SnV-Ls	0,205	0,326
Co-Gn and SnV-Li	0,011	0,959
Co-Gn and LsLi-HV	0,233	0,263
Co-Gn and SnV-Pog'	-0,080	0,702
Co-Gn and SnV-Pn	0,266	0,199

Co-Gn and A-Nperp	-0,036	0,865
Co-Gn and Pog-Nperp	-0,028	0,895
Co-A and SnV-Ls	0,213	0,307
Co-A and SnV-L	0,031	0,883
Co-A and LsLi-HV	0,216	0,300
Co-A and SnV-Pog'	-0,115	0,583
Co-A and SnV-Pn	0,150	0,475
Co-A and A-Nperp	0,217	0,297
Co-A and Pog-Nperp	-0,150	0,473
SnV-Ls and SnV-Li	0,764	<0,001***
SnV-Ls and LsLi-HV	0,060	0,775
SnV-Ls and SnV-Pog'	0,360	0,077
SnV-Ls and SnV-Pn	-0,170	0,416
SnV-Ls and A-Nperp	0,262	0,206
SnV-Ls and Pog-Nperp	0,125	0,551
SnV-Li and LsLi-HV	-0,598	0,002**
SnV-Li and SnV-Pog'	0,700	<0,001***
SnV-Li and SnV-Pn	-0,121	-0,563
SnV-Li and A-Nperp	0,182	0,384
SnV-Li and Pog-Nperp	0,176	0,400
LsLi-HV and SnV-Pog'	-0,632	0,001**
LsLi-HV and SnV-Pn	-0,032	0,878
LsLi-HV and A-Nperp	0,046	0,825
LsLi-HV and Pog-Nperp	-0,109	0,606
SnV-Pog' and SnV-Pn	-0,187	0,371
SnV-Pog' and A-Nperp	0,383	0,058
SnV-Pog' and Pog-Nperp	0,543	0,005**
SnV-Pn and A-Nperp	-0,218	0,296
SnV-Pn and Pog-Nperp	-0,161	0,442
A-Nperp and Pog-Nperp	0,749	<0,001***

*p<0.05; **p<0.01; ***p<0.001

APPENDIX D - Values found for cephalometric quantities

Sample	FNA	SNA	SNB	ANB	1.NA	1.NB
CT	86,39	93,58	87,25	6,33	17,64	32,11
CG	84,62	90,19	87,62	2,57	30,28	27,42
CC	92,28	83,21	81,12	2,09	27,38	30,11
CO	83,06	94,6	91,77	2,83	25,53	24,43
DBS	93,46	76,94	77,95	-1,02	32,05	16,86
FS	89,82	86,04	83,4	2,65	26,24	24,77
MS	93,94	85,93	87,8	-1,86	38,22	31,27
PPF	96,94	80,12	80,51	-0,39	31,28	26,27
RF	90,74	81,46	80,62	0,84	15,36	22,03
RR	90,61	80,42	79,65	0,77	29,26	25,58
RB	94,87	74,62	77,39	-2,77	36,05	21,9
RBC	90,57	77,35	75,24	-2,1	28,35	26,69
AFS	90,41	85,1	83,46	1,63	32,67	30,21
EDL	88,04	88,97	87,55	1,42	26,11	27,75
FS	92,03	87,32	86,96	0,36	27,27	27,78
FCO	90,82	80,88	78,32	2,57	15,89	32,81
LSL	91,26	84,51	85,19	-0,68	24,39	19,49
PJ	95,62	81,56	79,81	1,76	32,94	27,43
RR	89,25	83,25	80,12	3,12	24,12	29,01
RA	81,64	90,48	84,1	6,38	13,71	24,88
PZ	87,06	90,36	84,37	5,99	16,34	31,94
KBL	91,82	84,95	83,39	1,57	29,14	26,21
BS	87,21	89,94	87,12	2,82	24,68	26,99
GD	93,28	82,36	79,14	3,22	26,11	34,29
JCM	82,69	85,76	80,58	5,17	15,8	32,22
Average	89,94	84,80	82,82	1,81	25,87	27,22
DesvPd*	4,04	5,12	4,11	2,51	6,76	4,26
Minimum	81,64	74,62	75,24	-2,77	13,71	16,86
Maximum	96,94	94,6	91,77	6,38	38,22	34,29

Sample	FMA	FNP	Co-Gn	Co-A	Snper-Ls	Snperp-Li
CT	22,92	91,29	144,83	111,14	3,77	-0,09
CG	31,74	86,99	133,23	95,05	3,42	-0,31
CC	25,38	93,38	122,63	93,94	0,76	-3,24
CO	19,28	84,62	131,92	97,98	2,85	2,76
DBS	21,17	90,71	131,07	94,08	0,59	-1,57
FS	20,3	91,13	140,13	106,77	2,55	1,4

MS	26,75	90,23	130,69	91,55	1,94	0,28
PPF	28,68	94,4	143,33	100,02	4,27	0,98
RF	23,53	89,82	152,91	111,75	1,63	-1,67
RR	21,85	90,97	125,49	94,97	3,18	1,91
RB	25,6	90	150,31	104,75	2,39	-0,8
RBC	21,52	91,26	131,51	103,34	0,8	-0,86
AFS	18,36	91,42	131,83	99,77	0,13	-1,52
EDL	17,02	87,64	134,93	104,4	2,94	0,1
FS	21,24	91,08	143,61	106,15	1,24	-1,23
FCO	21,81	92,66	139,8	106,34	1,86	-0,48
LSL	22,97	88,91	137,43	98,42	0,22	-1,68
PJ	20,85	94,39	134,77	101,68	1,43	-0,95
RR	23,31	90,73	133,29	104,18	3,71	1,63
RA	20,36	86,54	145,28	110,84	1,34	-2,4
PZ	22,01	91,86	136,79	108,3	2,32	0,56
KBL	23,26	92,44	141,99	107,2	0,79	-1,89
BS	24,49	88,92	147,72	109,42	4,52	3,49
GD	24,64	95,89	143,18	115,98	2,87	-0,09
JCM	23,82	87,12	133,9	105,23	3,59	-0,41
Average	22,91	90,58	137,70	103,33	2,20	-0,24
DesvPd*	3,18	2,65	7,56	6,43	1,29	1,61
Minimum	17,02	84,62	122,63	91,55	0,13	-3,24
Maximum	31,74	95,89	152,91	115,98	4,52	3,49

Sample	LsLi-HV	Snperp-Pg	Pr-Sn	A-Nperp	Pog-Nperp
CT	3,86	-9,27	15,66	3,89	-2,95
CG	3,73	-5,09	16,02	5,32	6,37
CC	4	-11,55	16,9	-2,29	-6,82
CO	0,09	-0,04	14,96	6,51	11,03
DBS	2,16	-6,64	15,28	-3,57	-1,48
FS	1,15	-3,31	19,28	0,21	-2,52
MS	1,66	-4,68	16,18	-4,03	-0,48
PPF	3,29	-6,99	18,88	-7,49	-10,13
RF	3,3	-6,25	20,07	-0,85	0,43
RR	1,27	-4,62	20,17	-0,65	-2,03
RB	3,19	-6,8	19,37	-6,12	0
RBC	1,66	-7,1	18,1	-0,66	-2,71
AFS	1,65	-7,79	19,43	-0,44	-2,96
EDL	3,04	-4,76	15,53	2,2	4,75

FS	2,47	-9,01	22,44	-2,09	-2,25
FCO	2,34	-6,36	20,96	-0,93	-6,06
LSL	1,9	-3,83	19,64	-1,44	2,4
PJ	2,38	-8	19,18	-6,19	-9,65
RR	2,08	-3,79	17,83	0,83	-1,57
RA	3,74	-8	19,31	9,5	7,81
PZ	1,76	-1,92	16,91	3,07	-3,98
KBL	2,68	-6,68	14,35	-1,91	-5,35
BS	1,03	-3,11	17,66	3,17	2,48
GD	2,96	-8,96	16,61	-3,89	-13,07
JCM	4	-4,26	17,76	7,86	5,92
Average	2,46	-5,95	17,94	0,00	-1,31
DesvPd*	1,05	2,59	2,07	4,36	5,73
Minimum	0,09	-11,55	14,35	-7,49	-13,07
Maximum	4	-0,04	22,44	9,5	11,03

* Standard Deviation

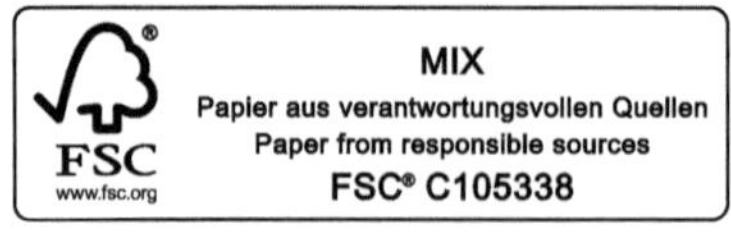

Printed by Books on Demand GmbH, Norderstedt / Germany